FOOD HERBS AND OILS

ALL NATURAL HOME REMEDIES

YVONNE P. JOHNSON, HHC

Copyright © 2015 by Yvonne P. Johnson All Right Reserved.

No part of this publication may be reproduced, distributed, or transmitted in any form or by any means, including photocopying, recording, or other electronic or mechanical methods, or by any information storage and retrieval system without the prior written permission of the publisher.

ISBN: 10:1511986107
ISBN-13:9781511986106

DISCLAIMER

All information is intended for your general knowledge only and is not a substitute for medical advice or treatment. You should seek medical advice before starting this or any other treatment regimen. The author makes no warranty, express or implied, regarding your individual results. The author disclaims any personal liability, for loss or risk incurred as a result of any information or advice contained herein, either directly or indirectly. All links are for informational purposes only and are not warranted for content, accuracy, or other implied or explicit purposes. All links were working at the time of this book release but may now have expired.

Thank You for purchasing my book: Food Herbs And Oils. As a bonus, I am offering a free eBook - Powerful Weight Loss Secrets And Tips: Download your free copy at:

http://www.bewealthybehealthybelieve.com

POWERFUL WEIGHT LOSS SECRETS AND TIPS

Lose The Fat and Gain A New Body

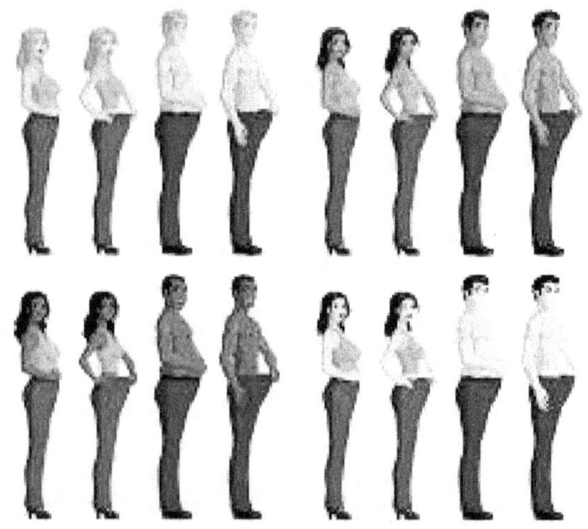

YVONNE P. JOHNSON, HHC

Lose The Fat and Gain A New Body

Sign up to download the **Free Weight Loss eBook and Free Newsletter** with more life changing health and fitness information at:

http://www.bewealthybehealthybelieve.com

TABLE OF CONTENTS

INTRODUCTION

Here's Good News… You Can Affect Your Health Positively With; Food, Herbs and Oils as Your Medicine!

Many of us have heard the ancient saying, "Let your medicine be your food, and food be your medicine" It's a wise saying by Hippocrates, the ancient Greek physician. The idea that our food can be our medicine is usually not included in the practice of modern medicine.

Did you know that herbal health care happens to be the oldest and most widely known form of medicine or therapy to mankind, used by many different cultures throughout the world? The World Health Organization (WHO) has estimated that about 80 percent of the world's population (approximately 4 billion people) is using some form of natural remedy as an aspect of primary health care.

In this modern world we live in today, there are many pollutants, the foods are being over processed and many preservatives are added to increase shelf life. These preservatives may be harmful to our health, especially when taken in large amounts. Most of the processed foods have lesser nutrients than foods in their natural state. Is it any wonder why most people are hoping for the intervention of natural remedies to improve their health?

Food, Herbs and Oils support the body's natural healing process and therefore; they are used for treatment or to bring back balance in a particular system in the body (they have proven therapeutic properties like boosting health, improving skin conditions, easing stress and generally benefiting the body and mind). Nature provides us with a wide range of extraordinary Foods and Herbs; they may be used in the form of extracts, tinctures, teas or even tablets.

All natural home remedies in this book will include the use of Food Herbs and Oils. An herb is either a plant or part(s) of a plant that is valued due to its medicinal, aromatic and savory qualities and abilities; they may be eaten or applied to the skin. When thinking of natural home remedies, picture nature as a cabinet full of medicine for most ailments.

Natural home remedies are a great way to treat aches, infections and pain from the comfort of your own home. Natural home remedies also have countless benefits over modern medicine and pharmaceutical drugs, some are highlighted below:

Natural Home Remedies-Are A Preventative Measure: Many prescription medications help to relieve lots of unpleasant symptoms that you're experiencing at the time but don't address the root cause. This makes the ache, infection or pain likely to resurface again and again. Natural home remedies work with your body's self-healing processes to target the source of the ailment and reduce the likelihood of future occurrences.

Natural Home Remedies-Don't Require A Prescription: Prescription medications are only available with a prescription from your doctor. Natural home remedies are much more accessible and can be prepared using herbs, fruits, spices, vegetables, oils and teas; which are widely available in health food and grocery stores, many of which you probably have in your house right now.

Natural Home Remedies-Are Multi-Functional: Prescription medications are designed to treat one specific ailment. Therefore, if you use prescription medications to treat multiple ailments, you'll have to purchase and consume specific drugs for each ailment which is both costly and inconvenient. The ingredients in natural home remedies can be used to treat a wide range of ailments and if you're suffering from multiple aches or infections, you can often prepare a single natural home remedy that targets them all.

Natural Home Remedies-Have Fewer Side Effects: Prescription medications often have a long list of unpleasant potential side effects with some of the most common including constipation, dizziness, drowsiness, nausea, vomiting and skin reactions. Natural home remedies on the other hand have little to no side effects, even when used on a regular basis.

Natural Home Remedies-Are Low Cost: Prescription medications require large amounts of research, testing and marketing and these all add considerably to their final cost. Natural home remedies don't have any of these added expenses and often cost a small amount to prepare.

Remember The Good News… You Can Affect Your Health Positively With; Food, Herbs and Oils as Your Medicine!

"Let food be thy medicine, and let thy medicine be food."

HIPPOCRATES

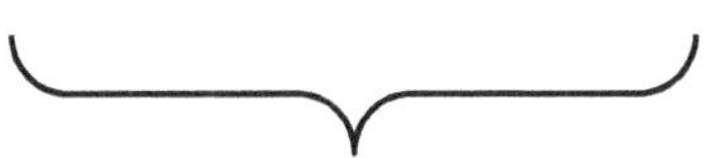

HOW TO USE THIS BOOK

ALL HOME REMEDIES IN THIS BOOK IS DIVIDED INTO FOUR (4) PARTS FROM A THRU Z

FOR EACH REMEDY YOU WILL GET:

1. An explanation of how the natural home remedy works.
2. A description of how to prepare the natural home remedy.
3. Tips and Variations for getting the most out of the natural home remedy.

Start enjoying all of the benefits with 95+ Natural Home Remedies that You Can Start Using Right Now!

PART 1: A THRU E

"Nature needs no remedy – she needs only an opportunity to exercise her own self-healing powers."

ANONYMOUS

ACID REFLUX

NATURAL HOME REMEDY

APPLE CIDER VINEGAR & MANUKA HONEY

HOW THE REMEDY WORKS

Acid reflux occurs when acidic gastric fluid moves up into the esophagus. Its symptoms include nausea, pain in the lower chest and a sour taste in the mouth. Most people experience these symptoms after eating a big meal or when lying down. A lot of people are often surprised that there are so many natural remedies that work fantastic for soothing the burn of heartburn and the upset stomach of indigestion.

This apple cider vinegar and manuka honey remedy helps to soothe acid reflux in the following ways:

1. **Apple Cider Vinegar:** Apple cider vinegar helps to treat acid reflux by stabilizing the acid levels in your stomach and promoting proper digestion.
2. **Manuka Honey:** Manuka honey is produced in New Zealand by bees that pollinate the native manuka bush. Honey has been used since ancient times to treat multiple conditions. Honey has an anti-inflammatory action that can quickly reduce pain and inflammation.

3. **Manuka honey** helps to treat acid reflux by repairing the tissues that line the esophagus and stomach which helps to limit any painful symptoms.

HOW TO PREPARE THE REMEDY

1. Add 1 tablespoon of apple cider vinegar and 1 teaspoon of manuka honey to a cup of hot water, mix well and drink.
2. Drink this remedy 30 minutes before each meal until the acid reflux subsides.

REMEDY VARIATIONS/TIP:

1. **Cabbage:** Eating cabbage can help to reduce and control the amount of acid that is produced in the stomach, therefore reducing acid reflux. Try raw cabbage (coleslaw) or fermented cabbage (sauerkraut) a delicious way to treat acid reflux.
2. **Ginger:** is an herb that can be added to the meals that you eat. Not only will it provide a nice taste, but it will also help to eliminate symptoms of acid reflux by promoting proper digestion.
3. **Pineapple:** You might think that pineapple would worsen acid reflux symptoms; it actually works to help in proper digestion due to its high level of enzymes.
4. **Raw Coconut Milk:** The burning sensation caused by acid reflux can be soothed by drinking a glass of raw coconut milk.

ACNE

NATURAL HOME REMEDY

BAKING SODA CINNAMON MANUKA HONEY & LEMON JUICE

HOW THE REMEDY WORKS

Acne is one of the most common skin diseases that affect about 85 percent of the population at some time in their life. Acne is a skin disorder that develops when the sebaceous glands of the skin become infected or inflamed and cause red pimples to develop on the surface of the skin.

Hormones also play a role, with hormone imbalances and changes often accompanying break-outs. Statistically, women are twice as likely as men to suffer adult acne, implicating a hormonal component to this often frustrating condition.

Sources also report that the prevalence of adult acne is on the rise. Women may notice a flare-up in their acne right before their menstrual period, which shows the role that hormones play in acne. In fact, male hormones are said to be the cause of acne in both genders, but women's hormonal levels change and fluctuate more than men's.

Teens and adults alike can have acne flare ups. The good news is you can get help from using natural remedies (teens and adults).

This baking soda, cinnamon, manuka honey and lemon juice remedy helps to treat acne in the following ways:

1. **Baking Soda:** Baking soda helps to treat acne by exfoliating your skin, unblocking your pores and getting rid of dead skin.
2. **Cinnamon:** Cinnamon is a powerful antioxidant that helps to repair the damage caused by acne.
3. **Manuka Honey:** Manuka honey helps to treat acne by reducing the buildup of bacteria in your pores and preventing inflammation on your skin.
4. **Lemon Juice:** Lemon juice helps to treat acne by drying out and disinfecting your skin.

HOW TO PREPARE THE REMEDY

1. Combine 5 tablespoons of manuka honey, 2 tablespoons of baking soda, and 2 tablespoons of lemon juice and 1 teaspoon of ground cinnamon in a bowl and mix well.
2. Apply the mixture to the acne for 5 minutes and then wash it clean with warm water. Use this remedy daily until the acne subsides.

REMEDY VARIATIONS/TIPS:

FACIAL CLEANSER: PINEAPPLE JUICE AND BAKING SODA

1. **Pineapple juice** contains enzymes that help treat acne. Mix 2 tablespoons of pineapple juice and enough baking soda to make a thin paste. Apply the mixture to the acne for 5 minutes and wash off with warm water.
2. **Facial Mask:** Masks are reputed to promote deep healing. They are left on the face for a period of time, and then rinsed off. You can make your own, here are some ideas:
3. **Cucumber:** Peel and seed a cucumber. Puree in a blender with enough milk or plain yogurt to make a thick liquid. Apply and leave on for about half an hour.
4. **Greek Yogurt and Lemon Juice:** Mix 1/4 cup plain Greek yogurt with 1 tablespoon lemon or grapefruit juice. Apply and leave on for 20-30 minutes; rinse.

TOPICAL TREATMENTS:

These are not intended to be rinsed off. Here are some to try.

1. **Aloe Vera:** Apply aloe vera juice to skin using a cotton ball.
2. **Cucumber:** Gently rub a slice of cucumber over acne-prone areas before bed.

Be gentle: lots of scrubbing and washing may irritate your skin more and worsen the acne.

ALLERGIES

NATURAL HOME REMEDY

NETTLE LEAF & PEPPERMINT

HOW THE REMEDY WORKS

Allergies are something that affects millions of people every single year with each season aggravating different types of allergies. While there are some people that are barely bothered by allergy symptoms, some only experience the symptoms of allergies on a seasonal basis. There are numerous others that experience them when they come in contact with dust particles, pets, and various other allergens. Shortly after exposure, allergy symptoms such as itchy watery eyes, coughing, sneezing, runny nose and skin rashes are often experienced. More people are taking advantage of the countless benefits that are provided with the use of natural herbs. Below is a list of some of the most popular herbs that are used by many allergy sufferers.

This nettle leaf and peppermint remedy helps to treat allergies in the following ways:

1. **Nettle Leaf:** Nettle leaf is a potent antihistamine (a substance that blocks the action of histamine - a chemical that gets

released during allergic reactions and causes many of their unpleasant symptoms).

2. **Peppermint:** Peppermint is an effective decongestant that can clear your nasal passages and also relieve any inflammation you may experience when suffering from allergies.

HOW TO PREPARE THE REMEDY

1. Add 1 tablespoon of dried nettle leaf and 1 tablespoon of dried peppermint to a cup of hot water and let it steep for 5 minutes.
2. After 5 minutes, strain the water into another cup using a fine mesh strainer and drink it.
3. Drink this remedy up to 4 times per day until the allergy symptoms subside.

REMEDY VARIATIONS/TIPS:

1. **Food Remedies**: Vitamin C: A natural antihistamine that can provide relief to allergy sufferers is vitamin C. It can be found in a variety of citrus fruits, berries, peppers, plums, spinach, and broccoli.
2. **Cinnamon:** Not only are the symptoms of allergies effectively reduced with the use of cinnamon, but the duration that they last is also reduced by a large amount. This is due to the natural antihistamine properties that are contained in cinnamon.

3. **Garlic:** The symptoms and irritations that allergies generally cause can be reduced with the natural antiviral properties of garlic.
4. **Licorice:** This herb is known for its effectiveness at decreasing inflammation that can occur with allergies.
5. **Parsley:** It is a well-known fact that parsley helps to promote the production and release of the natural antihistamines within the body that fight against bothersome allergy symptoms.
6. **Rosemary:** This herb is used by numerous people that suffer from asthma as well as the symptoms of allergies.

ANXIETY

NATURAL HOME REMEDY

CHAMOMILE OIL & LAVENDER OIL

HOW THE REMEDY WORKS

There are many people that experience the uneasiness, nervousness, stress, and worry that is commonly associated with anxiety. Excessive amounts of stress and anxiety can lead to a wide range of health conditions. This is why it is essential to take the steps needed to avoid situations that cause high levels of anxiety in your life. There are also some natural herbs that work very well at decreasing levels of anxiety.

This chamomile oil and lavender oil remedy helps to treat anxiety in the following ways:

1. **Chamomile Oil**: Chamomile oil has a soothing, relaxing effect and helps you to feel at ease. Chamomile is a sweet tasting herb that works wonders after a rough exhausting day at work. When used in a tea it is very effective for calming the nerves and soothing the mind. The effects of chamomile are extremely relaxing, and it also works great for an upset stomach.
2. **Lavender Oil:** Lavender oil is a natural relaxant and helps to eliminate feelings of anxiety.

HOW TO PREPARE THE REMEDY

1. Add 5 drops of chamomile oil and 5 drops of lavender oil to a hot bath and soak in it for up to 30 minutes.
2. Use this remedy every time you feel the symptoms of anxiety.

REMEDY VARIATIONS:

1. **Ginkgo biloba**: is also very helpful when used in a tea, and it provides a soothing sweet taste. This natural herb contains a high level of alkaloids that can help a great deal in improving the thoughts of a person's mind. A lot of people that drink ginkgo biloba tea quickly notice a reduction in the anxiety they feel, and it is replaced with a much more cheerful outlook. Another reason why numerous people enjoy ginkgo biloba tea is due to the beneficial increase of blood circulation that it promotes all throughout a person's body. Better blood circulation also results in a higher level of oxygen supplied to the brain.
2. **Kava Tea**: While there are many people that choose to use this herb in a tea, it can also be added to flavored waters, and taken with food at mealtime. Kava is a natural herb that has the ability to decrease levels of anxiety a person is experiencing, and it is accomplished naturally. As soon as a person begins to notice the dizziness, increased heart rate, and nervousness that are often associated with anxiety, using this natural herb can effectively reduce these negative feelings.

   The reason a lot of people choose to add kava to flavored water is because it can increase the benefits of kava. This is due to the magnesium, calcium, and derivatives of vitamin B complex contained in flavored water.

ARTHRITIS

NATURAL HOME REMEDY

GINGER MILK & TURMERIC

HOW THE REMEDY WORKS

Arthritis is a painful disorder which is characterized by inflammation in one or more of the joints. The symptoms of arthritis include pain, redness and swelling around the affected joints which can range from mild to severe. Reducing the pain of arthritis with natural remedies is Possible!

This ginger, milk and turmeric remedy helps to relieve the unpleasant symptoms of arthritis in the following ways:

1. **Ginger:** Ginger is a powerful anti-inflammatory that naturally reduces the joint inflammation associated with arthritis.
2. **Milk:** Milk keeps your joints healthy and protects them against inflammation.
3. **Turmeric:** Turmeric is also a natural anti-inflammatory which has been shown to be particularly effective at treating arthritis in clinical trials.

HOW TO PREPARE THE REMEDY

1. Add ½ teaspoon of ground ginger and ½ teaspoon of turmeric powder to a glass of warm milk mix well and drink it.
2. Drink this remedy daily to treat arthritis.

REMEDY VARIATIONS:

GINGER AND LEMON: Peel a fresh piece of ginger root and then cut about 12 to 15 pieces - each about the size of a quarter. Next, add the pieces of ginger to a small saucepan with about *2 cups of water and heat to boiling. *cup = 8 oz.

1. When the water comes to a boil, lower the heat to a low/medium simmer and simmer the ginger root pieces for about 15 minutes.
2. While the tea is simmering; squeeze the juice from 1/2 lemon into a cup. After 15 minutes, strain the tea pour into your cup with the lemon juice. If you want your tea to be spicier, take a couple of pieces of the ginger root and drop them into your tea cup. You can leave the ginger pieces in the cup for a stronger ginger tea.

BLACKSTRAP MOLASSES: Magnesium, potassium, and iron are a few of the minerals that are contained in blackstrap molasses. By dissolving just one tablespoon of molasses in a cup (6 ounces) of water you can benefit from relief of the pain arthritis causes, drink once daily.

TIPS:

EPSOM SALT (magnesium sulfate): Magnesium has both anti-inflammatory and anti- arthritic properties and it can be absorbed through the skin. Magnesium is one of the most important of the essential minerals in the body, and it is commonly deficient in the American diet. Try this remedy for arthritis: A hot bath of Epsom Salt. The heat of the bath can increase circulation and reduce the swelling of arthritis.

HOW TO PREPARE: Fill a bathtub with water as hot as you can stand. Add 2 cups of Epsom salts. Bathe for thirty minutes, adding hot water as necessary to keep the temperature warm. Do this daily, as often as you'd like to help relieve arthritis symptoms.

ASTHMA

NATURAL HOME REMEDY

EUCALYPTUS OIL & LAVENDER OIL

HOW THE REMEDY WORKS

Asthma is a breathing disorder that causes the airways to tighten and make breathing difficult or impossible. The symptoms of asthma include coughing, shortness of breath, tightness in the chest and wheezing. Asthma affects people of all ages, but it most often starts during childhood. In the United States, more than 25 million people are known to have asthma. About 7 million of these people are children.

This eucalyptus oil and lavender oil remedy helps to treat asthma in the following ways:

1. **Eucalyptus Oil:** Eucalyptus oil is a natural decongestant and helps to clear your airways, make breathing easier and prevent the buildup of mucus.
2. **Lavender Oil:** Lavender oil relives inflammation in your airways, helps them to widen and allows more air to get through.

HOW TO PREPARE THE REMEDY

1. Put 5 drops of eucalyptus oil and 5 drops of lavender oil on a paper towel and then place it on your pillow while you sleep.
2. When you wake up, discard the paper towel, add 5 drops of eucalyptus oil and 5 drops of lavender oil to a bowl of boiling water and breathe in the steam with deep breaths for 5 minutes.
3. Use this remedy daily to naturally treat asthma.

TIPS:

Stay away from substances that trigger your symptoms
Here are some common asthma triggers:

- Animals (pet hair or dander)
- Dust mites
- Chemicals in the air or in food
- Mold
- Pollen
- Tobacco smoke

Asthma attacks can last for minutes to days, and can become dangerous if the airflow is severely blocked.

Call 911 if you have any severe asthma symptoms.

BACK PAIN

NATURAL HOME REMEDY

ALMOND OIL & CAYENNE

HOW THE REMEDY WORKS

Back pain is something that affects millions of people around the world. Common causes of back pain include poor posture, a sedentary lifestyle and placing excessive strain on your back. Back pain can occur anywhere along the spine and can manifest as tightness, numbness or a sharp pain. If you feel pain in the back, which you believe is not an emergency; you should rest your back. When pain starts from common activates, it is often because you have over-exerted the joints, muscles, etc. When treating the problem at home, rest in a comfortable position. Lie on your back and place a pillow under your knees. You can also try resting on your back while placing your feet on your couch or chair. The knees should bend at a 90-degree angle. Roll a towel up and situated it so that it supports your neck.

This almond oil and cayenne remedy helps to relieve back pain in the following ways:

1. **Almond Oil:** Almond oil has analgesic properties and naturally soothes painful bones, joints and muscles when applied topically.
2. **Cayenne:** Cayenne contains high levels of capsaicin - a common ingredient in many topical pain relief creams which is one of the most effective natural solutions for fighting back pain.

HOW TO PREPARE THE REMEDY

1. Add 2 tablespoons of almond oil and 1 teaspoon of cayenne powder to a bowl and mix well.
2. Apply the mixture to the affected area of your back for 10 minutes and then wash it clean with warm water.
3. Use this remedy up to 3 times per day until the pain subsides.

TIP:

Back pain can emerge from various causes, yet when the pain is severe, one should seek medical advice immediately.

BAD BREATH

NATURAL HOME REMEDY

FENNEL SEEDS & LEMON JUICE

HOW THE REMEDY WORKS

Bad breath (Halitosis) is an unpleasant disorder that can be caused by eating certain types of foods, gum disease, smoking and other medical disorders. Halitosis is a frustrating problem that can easily be treated once it is known that dental problems are not at the root of the issue. Below is a list of some popular home remedies that are sure to provide you with the freshest breath ever.

This fennel seeds and lemon juice remedy helps to prevent bad breath in the following ways:

1. **Fennel Seeds:** Fennel seeds fight many of the common bacteria on the gums and tongue that cause bad breath.
2. **Lemon Juice:** The acid in lemon juice prevents the growth of bad breath causing bacteria in your mouth.

HOW TO PREPARE THE REMEDY

1. Add 1 tablespoon of lemon juice and 1 teaspoon of ground fennel seeds to a cup of boiling water, let it steep for 5 minutes and drink it.
2. Drink this remedy up to 4 times per day until the bad breath subsides.

REMEDY VARIATIONS/TIPS:

- Chew on fennel, dill, cardamom, or anise seeds. Anise, which tastes like black licorice, can kill the bacteria that grow on the tongue. Fennel, dill, and cardamom help mask the odor of halitosis. Chew on and savor the taste of mint leaves
- Eating apples promotes fresh breath
- Before brushing your teeth, use some hydrogen peroxide to rinse the mouth out
- Put a clove in your mouth and chew on it
- Dissolve some baking soda in water and use the mixture to gargle with
- Drinking pineapple juice can lick halitosis quickly.

TIPS: Use a tongue cleaner to prevent bad breath.
Your tongue can become coated with bacteria that ferment proteins, producing gases that smell bad. Scraping your tongue can dislodge these bacteria so you can rinse them away. A tongue cleaner is a thin, U-shaped piece of plastic or stainless steel with a blunted edge to remove coated bacteria from the surface of the tongue. The tongue cleaner will help eliminate bad breath at the source. If you are not already using a tongue cleaner…**Try it!**

BLACKHEADS

NATURAL HOME REMEDY

GREEN TEA & TEA TREE OIL

HOW THE REMEDY WORKS

Blackheads are a common skin disorder that occurs when the pores of your skin become blocked with bacteria and oil which causes small dark spots to form on the skin. Blackheads can affect people with any type of skin, but are generally more common in those with oily skin.

This green tea and tea tree oil remedy helps to get rid of blackheads in the following ways:

1. **Green Tea:** Green tea removes oil from the skin and unclogs blocked pores which help to treat existing blackheads and reduce the occurrence of blackheads in the future.
2. **Tea Tree Oil**: Tea tree oil opens up and disinfects your pores which help to clean and remove blackheads from your skin.

HOW TO PREPARE THE REMEDY

1. Crush 1 teaspoon of dry green tea leaves using a mortar and pestle.
2. Mix these ground dry green tea leaves with a small amount of water to form a paste.
3. Add 5 drops of tea tree oil to the paste.
4. Gently scrub the paste into the blackheads for 2 minutes and then wash them clean with warm water.
5. Use this remedy daily until the blackheads are gone.

Green tea is known for its antibacterial anti viral properties. The secret of green tea is its catechin polyphenols, particularly epigallocatechin (EGCG) which is a powerful antioxidants.

TIPS/Facts about Green Tea Health Benefits

Note: According to several studies green tea is one of the most effective home medicines:

- Helpful for those who have rheumatoid arthritis
- Reduce the risk of having hypertension and elevated blood pressure
- Reduces the cholesterol level in the body
- Increases metabolism
- Helps body to fight viruses and bacteria by improving the defense action of the immune system
- Reduces the process of thrombosis which helps reduce heart attacks and strokes
- Helps in reducing fatigue and stress due to its calming action
- Fights cardio vascular diseases.

BLOATING

NATURAL HOME REMEDY

CARAWAY SEEDS & FENNEL SEEDS

HOW THE REMEDY WORKS

Bloating is caused by the buildup of gas in the small intestine and can result in a visibly swollen stomach, belching, cramps and pain in the lower back.

This caraway seeds and fennel seeds remedy helps to treat bloating in the following ways:

1. **Caraway Seeds:** Caraway seeds have carminative properties and can help to remove intestinal gas from the body which eases bloating.
2. **Fennel Seeds:** Fennel seeds are an intestinal spasmolytic and help to relax the muscles in your intestinal tract and remove gas more quickly. Fennel seeds are incredibly effective and also start working very quickly. Simply chew slowly on a small amount of fennel seeds or put them in a cup of boiled, hot water.

HOW TO PREPARE THE REMEDY

1. Add 1 teaspoon of ground caraway seeds and 1 teaspoon of ground fennel seeds to a cup of boiling water, let it steep for 5 minutes and drink it.
2. Drink this remedy up to 4 times per day until the bloating subsides.

REMEDY VARIATIONS: Natural Remedy for Gas and Bloating

Baking Soda and Lemon: Baking soda and lemon juice form carbon dioxide, which is a natural digestive aid. You will find complete relief with this excellent gas and bloating remedy within about 20 minutes. Simply squeeze the juice of one lemon into a glass filled with half water then add a teaspoon of baking soda and mix. After the "fizz" has gone fill the rest of the glass with water, mix again then drink.

- For even better results it is recommended that you combine this remedy with **Apple Cider Vinegar.** Not only does this help to alleviate digestion and gas problems, it will help to increase your body's pH level, which is absolutely crucial for overall good health and longevity!

- **Grapes -** Grapes are one of nature's fruits that naturally help to prevent bloating. To help with bloating you can choose to drink grape juice or add grapes to your daily diet.

BRONCHITIS

NATURAL HOME REMEDY

GINGER & MANUKA HONEY

HOW THE REMEDY WORKS

Bronchitis is a very common condition; it is a disorder that develops when the mucous membranes in the bronchial tubes become inflamed. The symptoms of bronchitis include breathing problems, chest pain and congestion. Bronchitis occurs in people of all ages. But elderly people, infants, and young children are at higher risk for acute bronchitis than people in other age groups. The two main types of bronchitis are acute (short term) and chronic (ongoing).

Acute bronchitis is caused by a virus and causes the build-up of phlegm in the throat, coughing and wheezing, sore throat, fever and exhaustion. The same viruses that cause colds and the flu are the most common cause of acute bronchitis. Bacteria can sometimes cause acute bronchitis. Most cases of acute bronchitis go away within a few days. However, coughing may last for several weeks after the infection is gone. Chronic bronchitis is an ongoing, serious condition. It occurs if the lining of the bronchial tubes is constantly irritated and inflamed, causing a long-term cough with mucus. Repeatedly breathing in fumes that irritate and damage lung and airway tissues causes chronic bronchitis. Smoking is the major cause of the condition. Breathing in air pollution and dust or fumes from the environment or workplace also can lead to chronic bronchitis. Viruses or bacteria can easily infect the irritated bronchial tubes. If this happens, the condition worsens and lasts longer.

This ginger and manuka honey remedy helps to treat bronchitis in the following ways:

1. **Ginger:** Ginger's anti-inflammatory properties help to reduce the inflammation caused by bronchitis and relieve many of its symptoms.
2. **Manuka Honey**: Manuka honey is a powerful antiviral and can help to fight many of the viruses that cause bronchitis.

HOW TO PREPARE THE REMEDY

1. Add 1 teaspoon of ground ginger and 1 teaspoon of manuka honey to a cup of boiling water, let it steep for 5 minutes and drink it.
2. Drink this remedy up to 4 times per day until the bronchitis subsides.

Also See Remedy For Common Cold in Part 1

BURNS

NATURAL HOME REMEDY

COCONUT OIL & RAW POTATO

HOW THE REMEDY WORKS

While major burns require immediate medical attention to prevent permanent damage, natural remedies are a great solution for minor burns. There are three levels of burns:

- First-degree burns affect only the outer layer of the skin. They cause pain, redness, and swelling.
- Second-degree burns affect both the outer and underlying layer of skin. They cause pain, redness, swelling, and blistering. They are also called partial thickness burns.
- Third-degree burns affect the deep layers of skin. They are also called full thickness burns. They cause white or blackened, burned skin. The skin may be numb.

This coconut oil and raw potato remedy helps to soothe minor burns in the following ways:

1. **Coconut Oil:** Coconut oil is loaded with fatty acids and vitamin E which collectively help to soothe and refresh burnt skin.

2. **Raw Potato:** Raw potatoes help to cool and moisturize burns which limit the associated pain and discomfort.

HOW TO PREPARE THE REMEDY

1. Massage 1 tablespoon of coconut oil into the burnt skin for 1 minute.
2. After 1 minute, cut a slice of raw potato and rub it into the burn for another minute.
3. Use this remedy every couple of hours until the pain, redness and swelling from the burn subsides.

Remember - third-degree burns and second degree burns more than 2-3 inches wide require immediate medical care.

TIPS:

For little kitchen burns, run cold water over them, then apply a slice of onion to block the pain receptors. Onion juices have antibacterial properties that may help prevent infection. Another way to help relieve pain from a burn is to rub Garlic Oil onto a burn.

Serious burns need immediate medical care. Call your local emergency number or 911.

CHAPPED LIPS

NATURAL HOME REMEDY

COCONUT OIL MILK & ROSE PETALS

HOW THE REMEDY WORKS

Chapped lips develop when the skin on the lips dries out and can cause your lips to become cracked, flaky, red and sore.

This coconut oil, milk and rose petals remedy helps to treat chapped lips in the following ways:

1. **Coconut Oil:** Coconut oil is loaded with fatty acids and vitamin E. Coconut oil is a very effective moisturizer and can help to rehydrate chapped lips.
2. **Milk:** Milk has a soothing effect on the skin and can help to relieve the symptoms of chapped lips.
3. **Rose Petals:** Rose petals contain high amounts of vitamin C, a powerful antioxidant. Rose petals also contain various oils that help to lock moisture into the lips and stop them from drying out.

HOW TO PREPARE THE REMEDY

1. Take a handful of rose petals and rinse them in water.
2. Add the rose petals and 1 cup of milk to a small bowl, and then leave them to soak for 4 hours.
3. After 4 hours, add 1 tablespoon of coconut oil to the bowl and then blend all the ingredients into a smooth mixture using a hand blender.
4. Apply this mixture to your lips up to 3 times per day until they are smooth and moist.

TIP:

Coconut oil can be used alone as a lip balm.

COLD SORES

NATURAL HOME REMEDY

TEA BAGS

HOW THE REMEDY WORKS

Tea is one of the most well-known and widely used natural remedies in the world. It was originally used by the ancient Chinese as a medicinal beverage around 2700 BC and today many countries and cultures enjoy its natural health benefits. Tea is rich in a range of phytonutrients which make it highly effective at fighting viral infections. Cold sores are caused by the herpes simplex virus-1 (HSV-1) and by applying teabags to the affected area, the powerful plant based nutrients in tea can treat the virus and protect against its adverse effects.

HOW TO PREPARE THE REMEDY

Creating a natural cold sore remedy with teabags is very easy. Simply follow the instructions below to prepare the remedy:

1. Soak a teabag in warm water and allow it to cool.

2. Once it has cooled, hold the wet teabag against the cold sore for 10 minutes.

To get the most out of this teabag cold sore remedy, apply a fresh teabag to the cold sore every 2 hours. Use black or green teabags.

REMEDY VARIATIONS/TIPS:

If you want to speed up your cold sore recovery, try combining the teabag cold sore remedy with the natural cold sore remedies listed below:

1. **Hydrogen Peroxide:** Hydrogen peroxide disinfects and dries out cold sores. To treat your cold sore with hydrogen peroxide and teabags, follow the remedy as outlined above, then discard the teabag, dip a cotton ball in 3% hydrogen peroxide solution, apply it to the cold sore, leave it for 10 minutes and then wipe it clean.
2. **Ice:** Ice is a simple but effective natural cold sore treatment that can reduce pain, redness and swelling around the affected area. To treat your cold sore with ice and teabags, follow the remedy as outlined above, then discard the teabag and hold an ice cube against the cold sore for another 10 minutes.
3. **Lemon Balm**: Lemon balm is an essential oil with antiviral properties that can help heal cold sores faster. To treat your cold sore with lemon balm and teabags, follow the remedy as outlined above, then discard the teabag and directly apply 1-2 drops of lemon balm essential oil to the cold sore.

4. **Milk:** Milk contains many ingredients which fight the HSV-1 virus. To treat your cold sore with milk and teabags, follow the remedy as outlined above, then discard the teabag, soak a cotton ball in milk and hold it against the cold sore for 10 minutes.

COMMON COLD

NATURAL HOME REMEDY

CAYENNE FENUGREEK SEEDS LEMON JUICE & MANUKA HONEY

HOW THE REMEDY WORKS

The common cold is a viral infection that many people suffer from in the winter months. Its symptoms include a persistent cough, a runny nose, headaches and tiredness. While there are no known cures for the common cold, this cayenne, lemon juice, manuka honey and fenugreek seeds remedy can help soothe many of its symptoms in the following ways:

1. **Cayenne:** Cayenne is a powerful decongestant and pain reliever which can help ease the congestion, headaches and sore throat that often come with the common cold.
2. **Fenugreek** Seeds: Studies have shown that fenugreek seeds can relieve almost all the symptoms associated with the common cold.
3. **Lemon Juice:** Lemon juice contains high levels of vitamin C - a nutrient that strengthens your immune system and helps it fight the common cold.

4. **Manuka Honey:** Manuka honey's antiviral properties help your body recover from the common cold at a faster rate.

HOW TO PREPARE THE REMEDY

1. Add 2 teaspoons of lemon juice, 1 teaspoon of manuka honey, 1 teaspoon of ground fenugreek seeds and ½ teaspoon of cayenne powder to a cup of boiling water, let it steep for 5 minutes and drink it.
2. Drink this remedy up to 4 times per day until the symptoms of the common cold subside.

TIPS:

One of the best and healthiest ways for a person to fight against suffering the symptoms of the common cold is to build up the defenses of the body's immune system. One of the biggest advantages of providing the body with essential vitamins and minerals is it not only fights against the symptoms of the common cold, but it helps to prevent them as well. Below you will find some of the most beneficial vitamins that help a great deal in the treatment of the common cold and ward off its frustrating symptoms:

Vitamin A - Fighting the symptoms of the common cold can be helped tremendously by simply taking 50 to 100k IU of vitamin A for a period of no longer than 5 days at a time.

Vitamin C - Taking high levels of vitamin C that consist of at least 3000 milligrams each day can help a great deal in helping to prevent the common cold from even starting.

Vitamin E - There is a large amount of toxins that are produced naturally within a person's body when the immune system is fighting against an infection like the common cold. Taking vitamin E in combination with vitamin C is a great way to protect the body's cells from the damage and oxidation that these free radicals can cause. A good amount of vitamin E to take would be 400 IU. Not only is this vitamin beneficial for the common cold, it also fights against many other serious health conditions as well.

Zinc - In some studies zinc has proven to be very effective at fighting against the virus that causes the common cold. It is suggested that taking about 120 to 140 milligrams, which is between four and six zinc lozenges each day for approximately 5 days can effectively kill the cold virus.

There have been numerous tests that have proven just how beneficial vitamins can be to the human body. It has also been proven that they are especially beneficial when a person has contracted the virus that causes the common cold.

CONJUNCTIVITIS

NATURAL HOME REMEDY

CALENDULA

HOW THE REMEDY WORKS

Conjunctivitis (also known as pink eye) is an eye infection that causes your eyes to become inflamed and pink colored.
Its symptoms include a burning sensation in the eyes, excessive tear production and extreme sensitivity to light.

This calendula remedy helps to treat conjunctivitis in the following ways:

Calendula: Calendula fights the bacteria and viruses that cause conjunctivitis. This herb is soothing and reduces swelling and itching as well as inflammation. It is helpful in infections like conjunctivitis, irritation due to pollution, allergies and minor injuries. It is antiseptic.

Apply Calendula as a cold or warm compress or use as an eyewash.

1. If an allergy is the problem, a cool compress may feel better.
2. If the pinkeye is caused by an infection, then a warm, moist compress may soothe your eye and help reduce redness and

swelling. A warm, moist compress can spread infection from one eye to the other.

3. Remember to use a different compress for each eye.

HOW TO PREPARE THE REMEDY

1. Add 1 teaspoon of dried calendula to a cup of hot *distilled water* and let it steep for 5 minutes.
2. After 5 minutes, strain the water into another cup using a fine mesh strainer and allow it to cool.
3. Once the water has cooled, fill an eyebath with it and then wash the affected eye; or use a cold or warm compress.
4. Use this remedy up to 4 times per day until the conjunctivitis subsides.

TIPS:

Know when to see your healthcare provider:

- When, conjunctivitis is accompanied by moderate to severe pain in the eye(s).
- When, conjunctivitis is accompanied by vision problems, such as sensitivity to light or blurred vision that does not improve when any discharge that is present is wiped from the eye.
- When, conjunctivitis is accompanied by intense redness in the eye(s).

CONSTIPATION

NATURAL HOME REMEDY

FIGS & FLAX SEEDS

HOW THE REMEDY WORKS

Constipation is a frustrating digestive disorder that makes it difficult to pass stools. Constipation happens when bowel movements become less frequent and are more difficult. Although the time between bowel movements widely ranges from person to person, going longer than three days without any bowel movement is too long. This is because after three days the feces or stool will become harder and a lot more difficult to pass through the anal opening. If you experience any of the following symptoms for three months or longer it can mean that you are considered constipated:

1. Your stools are hard more than twenty five percent of the time
2. You have two or less bowel movements in a week
3. You strain during a bowel movement more than twenty five percent of the time
4. You have incomplete evacuation of your stool more than twenty five percent of the time

This figs and flax seeds remedy helps to relieve constipation in the following ways:

1. **Figs:** Figs are a natural laxative. They also contain high levels of fiber which helps to clear waste materials out of your body and ease the passing of stools.
2. **Flax Seeds:** Flax seeds are rich in fiber and healthy fats which boost your digestive system and help waste materials pass through your body.

HOW TO PREPARE THE REMEDY

1. Blend 1 large dried fig and 1 tablespoon of flax seeds in a blender until it forms a thick paste and then consume this mixture.
2. Use this remedy up to 4 times per day until the constipation subsides.

TIPS:

- Add more vegetables and fruits to your diet.
- Eat bran cereal and prunes.
- Drink two to four extra glasses of water each day, unless fluid restricted.
- If this doesn't help, talk with your healthcare provider or doctor.

COUGHS

NATURAL HOME REMEDY

CAYENNE MILK & TURMERIC

HOW THE REMEDY WORKS

A cough is a natural reflex that protects your lungs. Coughing helps clear your airways of lung irritants. Persistent coughs can be caused by a variety of factors including blockages in the windpipe, environmental irritants: (examples of irritants are cigarette smoke, air pollution, paint fumes and scented products). Also some people have coughs due to viral infections and allergens (examples of allergens are animal dander, dust, and mold, pollen from trees, grasses, and flowers).

This cayenne, milk and turmeric remedy helps to treat coughs in the following ways:

1. **Cayenne:** Cayenne naturally warms and soothes the lining of your throat which helps to reduce any irritation that may lead to coughing.
2. **Milk**: Milk contains a range of nutrients that help to moisturize your throat and prevent it from drying out.
3. **Turmeric:** Turmeric's antiviral and anti-inflammatory action helps to alleviate many of the irritants that cause coughing.

HOW TO PREPARE THE REMEDY

1. Add 1 teaspoon of turmeric and ½ teaspoon of cayenne powder to a glass of hot milk, mix well and drink it.
2. Drink this remedy up to 4 times per day until the cough disappears.

Also See Remedy For Allergies In Part 1

CRAMPS

NATURAL HOME REMEDY

CLOVE OIL & ICE

HOW THE REMEDY WORKS

Cramps are rapid, uncontrollable muscle contractions that are often characterized by a sharp pain in the affected muscles. Cramps may involve all or part of one or more muscles. The cramping muscle may feel hard or bulging. The most common muscle groups are: Back of leg/calf - Back of thigh (hamstrings) and Front of thigh (quadriceps). Muscle cramps are common and often occur when a muscle is overused or injured. Muscle strain or simply holding a position for a prolonged period of time may result in a muscle cramp. Exercising when you haven't had enough fluids (dehydration) or when you have low levels of minerals such as potassium or calcium can also make you more likely to have a muscle spasm. In many cases, however, the exact cause of a muscle cramp isn't known.

This clove oil and ice remedy helps to treat cramps and reduce the risk of them coming back in the following ways:

1. **Clove Oil:** Clove oil helps the muscles to relax and can loosen up cramped muscles.
2. **Ice**: Ice provides instant pain relief from cramps.

HOW TO PREPARE THE REMEDY

1. Wrap 4 ice cubes in a small towel and hold it against the cramped muscles for 10 minutes.
2. After 10 minutes, massage 1 tablespoon of clove oil into the cramped muscles for 5 minutes and then wash it clean with warm water.
3. Use this remedy every couple of hours until the cramp subsides.

TIPS:

1. Drink plenty of fluids while exercising.
2. Increase your potassium intake (orange juice and bananas are great sources of potassium).

Remember - muscle cramps are common and may be stopped by stretching the muscle.

DANDRUFF

NATURAL HOME REMEDY

COCONUT OIL & EXTRA VIRGIN OLIVE OIL

HOW THE REMEDY WORKS

Dandruff is one of the most common chronic scalp disorders around. Its symptoms include dry, flaky skin, an itchy scalp and red rashes on the scalp. It's good to know that dandruff is not contagious and hardly ever serious; however it can be embarrassing and difficult to treat.

This coconut oil and extra virgin olive oil remedy helps to treat dandruff in the following ways:

1. **Coconut Oil:** Coconut oil has a moisturizing effect on the scalp and helps to prevent dry skin and any of the unpleasant associated symptoms.
2. **Extra Virgin** Olive Oil: Extra virgin olive oil is another potent natural moisturizer that also contains high levels of skin boosting vitamin E. It helps to keep the scalp healthy and dandruff free.

HOW TO PREPARE THE REMEDY

1. Warm ¼ cup of coconut oil and ¼ cup of extra virgin olive oil in a saucepan and mix it well.
2. Massage the mixture into your scalp thoroughly, and then wrap your hair in a towel for 30 minutes.
3. After 30 minutes, remove the towel, comb your hair thoroughly and then wash it. Use this remedy 3 times per week until the dandruff disappears.

Also See Remedy For Dry Scalp In Part 1

DEPRESSION

NATURAL HOME REMEDY

CARDAMOM & ST JOHN'S WORT

HOW THE REMEDY WORKS

Depression is an emotional disorder that causes constant feelings of dejection, sadness and despair. While serious depression often requires professional therapy, this cardamom and St John's wort remedy can also help treat depression in the following ways:

1. **Cardamom:** Cardamom is a natural antidepressant and can help lift your mood and make you feel more energized.
2. **St John's Wort:** St John's wort is one of the most effective natural treatments for depression and can alleviate many of the common symptoms associated with depression.
3. **St John's Wort** is an herb that has been known for many years to be very effective for minimizing feelings of depression and anxiety. If you take prescription drugs, it is very important to talk with your doctor prior to using this herbal treatment, as it can cause an interference with some prescription drugs.

HOW TO PREPARE THE REMEDY

1. Add 1 teaspoon of cardamom powder and 1 teaspoon of St John's wort to a cup of hot water and let it steep for 5 minutes.
2. After 5 minutes, strain the water into another cup using a fine mesh strainer and drink it.
3. Drink this remedy daily to treat depression.

TIP:

Exercise regularly: Exercises can release serotonin which is able to produce a natural high. This high can be enough to turn things around. It will lift you up from your gloomy state, and help you combat depression effectively.

DIABETES

NATURAL HOME REMEDY

BITTER GOURD & CINNAMON

HOW THE REMEDY WORKS

Diabetes is a health disorder where your body struggles to properly regulate your blood glucose levels. Diabetes is when your blood glucose, also called blood sugar, is too high. Blood glucose is the main type of sugar found in your blood and your main source of energy. Glucose comes from the food you eat and is also made in your liver and muscles. Your blood carries glucose to all of your body's cells to use for energy.
The three main types of diabetes are Type 1, Type 2, and Gestational Diabetes.

People can develop diabetes at any age; both men and women can develop diabetes. According to NIDDK - National Institute of Diabetes and Digestive and Kidney Diseases, symptoms for type 1 diabetes usually come on very rapidly whereas symptoms for type 2 diabetes may develop gradually over time. There are similar warning signs that overlap with type 1 and type 2 diabetes. But there are also symptoms that are specific to each type of the disease.

Type 1 Diabetes - Symptoms for type 1 diabetes can include:

- An increased thirst that is not satisfied after drinking extra fluids
- A frequent need to urinate (more than normal)
- A dry or fuzzy feeling inside the mouth
- Unexplained and sudden weight loss
- Feeling light-headed, weak or dizzy
- Sight problems such as blurry vision

Type 2 Diabetes - Symptoms for type 2 diabetes can include:

- Sharp or numbing pain in the legs
- Cuts or bruises that take a long time to heal
- Recurrent yeast infections
- Sight problems such as blurry vision
- An increased thirst that is not satisfied after drinking extra fluids
- A frequent need to urinate (more than usual)

Gestational Diabetes is a type of diabetes that develops only during pregnancy. Overweight or obese women have a higher chance of gestational diabetes. Also, gaining too much weight during pregnancy may increase your likelihood of developing gestational diabetes.

This bitter gourd and cinnamon natural remedy helps to treat diabetes in the following ways:

1. **Bitter Gourd:** Bitter gourd lowers your blood glucose levels and boosts the secretion of insulin (a hormone that helps to control blood glucose levels in your body).
2. **Note:** When a person consumes the juice found in this vegetable while having an empty stomach, it works very well at lowering high levels of blood glucose. This is due to the anti-diabetic properties that work much like insulin that are found in the juice of bitter melon.
3. **Cinnamon**: Cinnamon promotes healthy blood glucose levels in diabetics when used on a daily basis.

HOW TO PREPARE THE REMEDY

1. Extract the juice from 4 bitter gourds using a juicer.
2. Dilute the bitter gourd juice with water at a ratio of 3:1.
3. Add 1 teaspoon of ground cinnamon to the diluted bitter gourd juice, mix well and drink it.
4. Drink this remedy daily each morning before eating to manage your diabetes.

REMEDY VARIATIONS:

Below is a list of several different natural remedy options that can help to reduce and maintain healthy blood sugar levels:

- **Cayenne pepper:** When it is taken on a daily basis, approximately 5 grams of cayenne pepper has the ability to lower a person's blood sugar levels.

- **Natural sweeteners:** To reduce sugar intake and be able to more easily maintain blood sugar levels, natural sweeteners such as Stevia can be used in the place of regular sugar. Another benefit is there are no calories to worry about with Stevia.
- **Onion and garlic:** When used on a regular basis onion and garlic have both proven to effectively maintain healthy levels of blood sugar. Whether they are eaten boiled or raw, onions contain just the right level of APDS or allyl propyl disulphide, which prevents the liver from breaking insulin down. This is also a substance that promotes healthier levels of insulin production within the body.
- **Blueberries**: Consuming blueberries is a great way for diabetes sufferers to reduce high blood glucose levels. A delicious drink can also be made – add a teaspoon of blueberry tea leaves or teabag into a cup of hot water let it steep 3-4 minutes, remove leaves or bag and drink around three cups daily.
- **Omega 3:** This is a natural substance that is extremely effective at reducing and maintaining blood sugar levels. Large amounts of omega 3 can be found in fish products like cod liver oil and salmon.

TIP:

The above remedies work best along with diet and exercise.

Make sure you talk with your doctor before starting any self treatment for diabetes.

DIAPER RASH

NATURAL HOME REMEDY

CORNSTARCH & WHITE VINEGAR

HOW THE REMEDY WORKS:

Diaper rash is characterized by dry, inflamed skin around the buttocks and diaper area. Diaper rash is often related to wet or infrequently changed diapers, skin sensitivity, and chafing. It usually affects babies, though anyone who wears a diaper regularly can develop the condition.

This cornstarch and white vinegar remedy helps to treat diaper rash in the following ways:

1. **Cornstarch:** Cornstarch absorbs moisture from the baby's diaper and reduces risk of diaper rash.
2. **White Vinegar:** White vinegar helps to neutralize the urine in your baby's diaper and protects against the inflammation that can lead to diaper rash.

HOW TO PREPARE THE REMEDY

1. Add 1 teaspoon of white vinegar to 1 cup of water, mix well and use this mixture to wash your baby's bottom when you change their diaper.
2. Dry your baby's bottom with a towel, then sprinkle 1 tablespoon of cornstarch on their bottom and put the fresh diaper in place.
3. Use this remedy every time you change your baby's diaper until the rash is gone.

TIPS:

- **Witch hazel** is an astringent produced from the bark and leaves of the witch hazel shrub. Witch hazel has been used for many centuries for medicinal purposes.

- **Witch hazel** has also been proven to be an effective diaper rash remedy. Apply witch hazel extract on the affected areas using a cotton ball. Witch hazel soothes and heals diaper rash faster than most diaper rash topical treatments.

DRY EYES

NATURAL HOME REMEDY

CUCUMBER & LAVENDER OIL

HOW THE REMEDY WORKS

Dry eyes are a common but irritating disorder that causes your eyes to become dry and itchy. Dry eyes occur when the eye does not produce tears properly, or when the tears are not of the correct consistency and evaporate too quickly. Dry eyes can be a temporary or chronic condition: Dry eyes can make it more difficult to perform some activities, such as using a computer or reading for an extended period of time. Dry eye symptoms may include any of the following:

- Eye fatigue
- Stinging or burning of the eye
- Sandy or gritty feeling as if something is in the eye
- Pain and redness of the eye
- Episodes of blurred vision
- Uncomfortable contact lenses

Dry eyes can occur at any age, but elderly people frequently experience dryness of the eyes. According to the National Eye Institute nearly five million Americans 50 years of age and older are estimated to have dry eyes.

This cucumber and lavender oil natural remedy helps to treat dry eyes in the following ways:

1. **Cucumber**: Cucumber is over 95% water and contains a range of nutrients that help to hydrate your eyes.
2. **Lavender Oil**: Lavender oil can help reduce the itchiness that comes with dry eyes.

HOW TO PREPARE THE REMEDY

1. Add 4 drops of lavender oil to a bowl of warm water, stir the water, dip a small, clean cloth into the water, drain the excess water from the cloth and then place the cloth over your closed eyes for 5 minutes.
2. After 5 minutes, remove the cloth and place 2 fresh cucumber slices on your closed eyes for 5 minutes.
3. After 5 minutes, remove the cucumber slices, dip the cloth into the lavender oil and warm water mixture again, drain the excess water from the cloth and wipe your closed eyes. Use this remedy every time your eyes start to feel dry.

TIP:

Allow your eyes to rest when performing activities that require you to use your eyes for long periods of time.

DRY SCALP

NATURAL HOME REMEDY

BANANA & SESAME SEED OIL

HOW THE REMEDY WORKS

Dry scalp can be caused by a variety of factors and results in your scalp becoming excessively dry, itchy and sore.

This banana and sesame seed oil remedy helps to treat dry scalp in the following ways:

1. **Banana:** Banana contains a variety of oils and nutrients that moisturize your scalp.
2. **Sesame Seed Oil**: Sesame seed oil hydrates, soothes and repairs dry skin on the scalp.

HOW TO PREPARE THE REMEDY

1. Warm ½ cup of sesame seed oil in a saucepan and combine it with 2 mashed bananas.

2. Massage the mixture into your scalp thoroughly, and then wrap your hair in a towel for 30 minutes.
3. After 30 minutes, remove the towel, comb your hair thoroughly and wash it.
4. Use this remedy 3 times per week until scalp is normal.

Also See Remedy For Dandruff in Part 1

DRY SKIN

NATURAL HOME REMEDY

EXTRA VIRGIN OLIVE OIL & MILK

HOW THE REMEDY WORKS

Dry skin is a very common skin condition characterized by a lack of appropriate amount of water and natural skin oil in the layer of the skin called the epidermis. (epidermis is the upper or outer layer of the two main layers of cells that make up the skin). Dry skin can occur at any age and for many reasons. The signs and symptoms of dry skin are:

- Rough, scaly, or flaking skin.
- Itching.
- Gray, ashy skin in people with dark skin.
- Cracks in the skin, which may bleed if severe.
- Chapped or cracked lips.

Dry skin may be a mild, temporary condition lasting a few days to weeks. Dry skin may also become a more severe, long-term skin problem for some.

This extra virgin olive oil and milk natural remedy helps to treat dry skin in the following ways:

1. **Extra Virgin Olive Oil**: Extra virgin olive oil's moisturizing properties and skin boosting antioxidants help to treat dry skin.
2. **Milk:** Milk contains many vitamins and minerals that promote healthy, moist skin.

HOW TO PREPARE THE REMEDY

1. Apply a thin layer of extra virgin olive oil to the dry skin for 30 minutes.
2. After 30 minutes, warm some milk in a saucepan, soak a cloth in the warm milk and apply the soaked cloth to the dry skin for 5 minutes.
3. After 5 minutes, wash the dry skin clean with warm water.
4. Use this remedy daily until the dry skin subsides.

REMEDY VARIATION/TIP:

Some of the most effective (and least expensive) moisturizers are petroleum jelly (vaseline) and mineral oil, because they contain no water; they are best used while the skin is still damp from bathing, to seal in the moisture.

EAR INFECTION

NATURAL HOME REMEDY

APPLE CIDER VINEGAR & EXTRA VIRGIN OLIVE OIL

HOW THE REMEDY WORKS

Although both children and adults have been known to suffer from painful ear aches, it is a problem that occurs much more frequently in young children. This is a problem that often arises when the delicate structures that make up the ear become infected. When this happens it can be extremely painful and can result in the formation of pus. It can happen any time, but the winter months are a common time of the year that many children suffer from the symptoms of ear aches and ear infections. Pus will often form when an ear infection becomes severe.

To avoid permanent damage it is imperative to have serious ear infections treated as soon as possible. There are also other symptoms that often accompany severe ear aches, such as a fever and a cough. It is important to never use natural remedies in place of professional medical care. However, the following are some effective herbal remedies that can help much before you're able to get to the doctor.

This apple cider vinegar and extra virgin olive oil remedy helps to treat ear infections in the following ways:

1. **Apple Cider Vinegar:** Apple cider vinegar directly combats many of the viruses that cause ear infections.
2. **Extra Virgin Olive Oil:** Extra virgin olive oil helps to clear the built up wax in your ears that often causes ear infections.

HOW TO PREPARE THE REMEDY

1. Warm 2 tablespoons of extra virgin olive oil and 1 teaspoon of apple cider vinegar in a saucepan and mix it well.
2. Lie on a towel on your left side and grab a cloth, and then use a dropper to fill your right ear with the mixture and leave it for 10 minutes.
3. After 10 minutes, place the cloth over your right ear, turn so that the mixture drains onto the cloth and then rinse the cloth.
4. Continue How To Prepare The Remedy (ear infection right side).
5. Lie on the towel on your right side and keep hold of the cloth, then use the dropper to fill your left ear with the mixture and leave it for 10 minutes.
6. After 10 minutes, place the cloth over your left ear, turn so that the mixture drains onto the cloth and then rinse the cloth.
7. Use this remedy up to 2 times per day until the ear infection subsides.

REMEDY VARIATIONS:

Also try the below remedies for Ear Infections:

1. **Fenugreek:** Mixing a small amount of cow's milk with fenugreek works well as a pain reliever for ear infections, and can be placed directly into the affected ear.

2. **Ginger extract:** This is an herbal extract that can be heated and placed directly into the affected ear, providing a great amount of pain relief.

TIP:

Remember: Ear infections are painful and can affect your balance, hearing and reflexes. If your ear pain increases; even with the above home remedies treatment, call your doctor or healthcare provider without delay.

ECZEMA

NATURAL HOME REMEDY

COLLOIDAL OATMEAL, EPSOM SALT & LAVENDER OIL

HOW THE REMEDY WORKS

Eczema is a common skin disorder where patches of the skin become cracked, dry, itchy and inflamed.

This Epsom salt, oatmeal and lavender oil remedy helps to treat eczema in the following ways:

1. **Colloidal Oatmeal**: Colloidal oatmeal is a powerful anti-inflammatory that can soothe any skin affected by eczema. Oatmeal bath is a technique that has been used by numerous people for quite some time. It is easy, inexpensive, and it is very effective at reducing inflammation.
2. **Epsom Salt:** Epsom salt is another strong natural anti-inflammatory that can relieve and repair any skin that is affected by eczema.
3. **Lavender Oil:** Lavender oil cleanses and soothes any skin that is affected by eczema.

HOW TO PREPARE THE REMEDY

1. Add 10 drops of lavender oil, 1 cup of colloidal oatmeal and 1 cup of Epsom salt to a hot bath and soak in it for up to 30 minutes.
2. Use this remedy up to 3 times per week until the eczema subsides.

REMEDY VARIATIONS:

1. **Virgin coconut oil:** The moisturizing effect that can be obtained from virgin coconut oil is amazing, which makes it very effective for healing itchy dry skin. To benefit from smooth soft skin, it is essential to only use the virgin coconut oil selection. This is because after the oil has gone through the process of refining, many of the healing properties are lost. Some other oils that also contain great healing properties include grape seed oil, castor oil, and avocado oil.
2. **Natural soaps:** It is important to stay completely away from soaps that contain perfumes and chemicals, as they tend to only aggravate flare-ups of eczema. Instead, choose soaps and moisturizers that only contain pure and natural ingredients.
3. **Pastes:** There are quite a few natural items that can be used to make a paste that works wonders for soothing the discomfort often caused by eczema.
4. **Nutmeg** - Adding a small amount of water to nutmeg to form a paste can be applied to eczema flare-ups to obtain fast soothing relief.

5. **Mango** - For soothing comfort, the pulp of mango can be boiled in water for approximately thirty minutes. Then, allow it to cool and apply directly to the area of the skin that's affected.
6. **Aloe Vera** - The use of Aloe Vera can provide soothing relief very quickly. Simply break open a small piece of Aloe Vera and apply the substance on the affected area.
7. **Papaya seeds** - Taking some papaya seeds to mash up and apply to eczema flare-ups is a great technique that helps tremendously with itching.
8. **Vitamin supplements**: Skin that becomes dry and damaged from flare-ups of eczema will heal much faster when you take vitamin supplements. A few vitamin supplements that contain anti-oxidant properties that promote fast healing are vitamins C and vitamin E.
9. **Moisturizers** - Just as with soaps, you will want to only use moisturizers that do not contain harsh chemicals and fragrances. It is best to only use products that contain pure and natural ingredients.

TIP:

Take Luke warm baths: When you are suffering from eczema flare-ups, it is important to only use lukewarm water to run your bath. The idea is to keep the skin adequately moisturized and the use of hot water will only cause the skin to become even dryer.

EDEMA

NATURAL HOME REMEDY

EPSOM SALT & GRAPEFRUIT OIL

HOW THE REMEDY WORKS

Edema (also known as water retention) is a disorder that causes swelling in various areas of the body, due to the accumulation of excessive fluid in the tissues. Edema usually occurs in the feet, ankles and legs, but it can involve your entire body. Pregnant women and older adults often get edema, but it can happen to anyone.

This Epsom salt and grapefruit oil remedy helps to treat edema in the following ways:

1. **Epsom Salt:** Epsom salts contain magnesium sulfate - a mineral that helps to reduce swelling.
2. **Grapefruit Oil:** Grapefruit oil also naturally reduces the swelling associated with edema.

HOW TO PREPARE THE REMEDY

1. Add 10 drops of grapefruit oil and 2 cups of Epsom salt to a hot bath and soak in it for up to 30 minutes.
2. Use this remedy up to 3 times per week until the edema subsides.

TIPS:

To help keep the swelling down try the below tips:

- Try limiting your salt intake.
- Elevate your legs when you are sitting or lying down.
- If you have edema of the legs, wear support stockings.
- Don't sit or stand for long periods of time without moving around.

ENERGY

NATURAL HOME REMEDY

APPLE, MATCHA GREEN TEA & SPINACH

HOW THE REMEDY WORKS

Energy is needed for the various functions like maintenance of growth, daily activities, exercise and many other movements or functions that are often taken for granted. Forget about energy drinks and coffee. It is possible to increase energy naturally, and have a healthy steady supply to get you through each day. By adjusting your personal eating, sleeping and exercise patterns, you can fight tiredness and boost your energy level fast and naturally.

This apple, matcha green tea and spinach remedy boosts your energy in the following ways:

1. **Apples:** Apples are rich in energy boosting carbohydrates and phytonutrients.
2. **Matcha Green Tea:** Matcha green tea contains caffeine and L-Theanine which collectively provide you with a sustained energy boost.
3. **Spinach**: Spinach is loaded with B vitamins which support energy production in your body.

HOW TO PREPARE THE REMEDY

1. Blend 1 apple, 1 cup of apple juice, 1 cup of spinach and 1 teaspoon of matcha green tea in a blender until smooth and then drink it.
2. Drink this remedy every time you need an energy boost.

TIPS:

Your body needs fuel to keep your energy levels up.

1. **Drink more water.** Dehydration causes fatigue, so keep your body hydrated throughout the day.
2. **Eat more protein**. Insufficient protein is a common reason for fatigue. Pack some almonds and nuts for a quick and convenient protein snack or have a hard-boiled egg for breakfast.
3. **Watch out for excess sugar**. Excess sugar causes fluctuating blood sugar levels, which can result in plummeting energy levels. Try to decrease all forms of refined sugars, including the "hidden sugars" in low-fat foods.
4. **Maintain a steady supply of nutrients to your body and increase your long-term energy levels.** Incorporate proteins, whole grains, high-fiber vegetables and nuts into your diet to keep blood sugar levels balanced.
5. **Make sure your bigger meals** are in the middle of the day rather than at night. Your digestion is naturally tuned to be more effective during the day, allowing your body to break down food for energy more effectively.

ERECTILE DYSFUNCTION

NATURAL HOME REMEDY

CARROT & POMEGRANATE JUICE

HOW THE REMEDY WORKS

Erectile dysfunction (also known as ED) is a health disorder that is believed to affect around 50% of men at some point in their lives. It is a very normal thing for a man to experience changes in the functioning of their penis, such as the length of time it takes to achieve a full and satisfactory erection.
However, if the problem is persistent then there may be other problems at hand such as an emotional or physical problem. ED (erectile dysfunction) can be the total inability of being able to achieve an erection, a tendency to only sustain a brief erection, or an inconsistent ability to achieve a full erection.

This carrot and pomegranate juice remedy helps to treat ED in the following ways:

1. **Carrot:** Carrot boosts sex hormone levels, enhances male libido and protects against impotence.
2. **Pomegranate Juice:** pomegranate juice is very high in Vitamin C and rich in antioxidants, and also increases the blood flow to the genital area.

3. Pomegranate juice increases testosterone levels in men and can help you overcome ED.

HOW TO PREPARE THE REMEDY

1. Blend 1 carrot and 1 cup of pomegranate juice in a blender until smooth and then drink it.
2. Drink this remedy daily to treat and protect against ED.

TIPS:

Tip: Only drink fresh carrot and pomegranate juice, without preservatives and sugar free.

With ED the first step to treating the problem is to find out what is causing it. The best doctor to discuss this problem with is an urologist or your primary care doctor. The best part is that this issue is fully treatable and fixable with the correct approach.

PART 2: F THRU J

"If we could give every individual the right amount of nourishment and exercise, not too little and not too much, we would have found the safest way to health."

Hippocrates

FATIGUE

NATURAL HOME REMEDY

BASIL OIL & EUCALYPTUS OIL

HOW THE REMEDY WORKS

Fatigue is one of the most common health complaints and can leave you feeling drained, exhausted and lacking in energy. Fatigue is caused by several factors such as viral infection, overexertion and lack of sleep. The feeling of exhaustion is usually relieved after the person gets some rest. If a person suffers from fatigue for extended periods of time, usually more than 6 months, he/she may be suffering from chronic fatigue syndrome.
Aside from herbal remedies, living a healthy life and having a balanced, healthy diet can help the individual overcome the symptoms of chronic fatigue syndrome. Fruits and vegetables provide the body with the important vitamins and minerals to keep the immune system strong.

This basil oil and eucalyptus oil remedy helps to fight fatigue in the following ways:

1. **Basil Oil:** Basil oil stimulates your mind and boosts your concentration levels when you feel tired.

2. **Eucalyptus Oil:** Eucalyptus oil is invigorating and energizing and naturally combats fatigue.

HOW TO PREPARE THE REMEDY

1. Add 5 drops of basil oil and 5 drops of eucalyptus oil to a hot bath then soak in it for up to 30 minutes.
2. Use this remedy every time you feel fatigued.

Also See Remedy For Energy In Part 1

FEVER

NATURAL HOME REMEDY

BASIL & GINGER

HOW THE REMEDY WORKS

A Fever is the temporary increase in the body's temperature. Most fevers develop as the result of illness and infection and can lead to dehydration, headaches, sweating and weakness.

This basil and ginger remedy helps to treat fevers in the following ways:

1. **Basil:** Basil fights inflammation and infection and can directly treat many causes of fevers.
2. **Ginger:** Ginger is a natural antiviral and can combat the viruses that lead to fevers.

HOW TO PREPARE THE REMEDY

1. Add 1 teaspoon of ground basil and 1 teaspoon of ground ginger to a cup of boiling water, let it steep for 5 minutes and drink it.

2. Drink this remedy up to 4 times per day until the fever subsides.

TIPS:

1. To help cool someone with a fever, try a lukewarm bath or a sponge bath.
2. Drink plenty of fluids (water) and rest.

FIBROIDS

NATURAL HOME REMEDY

DANDELION & MILK THISTLE

HOW THE REMEDY WORKS

Fibroids are non-cancerous tumors which develop in and around the uterus. They are made up of fibrous and muscle tissue and can vary in size. Many women who have fibroids are unaware of their presence as they do not experience any symptoms. In most cases fibroids are detected during routine gynecological checkups.

Many women tolerate day to day life experiencing a wide range of symptoms typical of fibroids without actually knowing this is what they have. Heavy bleeding that follows the monthly cycle, severe cramps and lower back pain, increased fatigue and forgetfulness, cramps, headaches and general unease, are just some of the many symptoms that come with fibroids.

This dandelion and milk thistle remedy helps to treat fibroids in the following ways:

1. **Dandelion:** Dandelion detoxifies the liver and removes excess estrogen from the body which reduces your risk of developing fibroids.
2. **Milk** Thistle: Milk thistle helps to balance hormone levels in your body and prevents fibroids.

HOW TO PREPARE THE REMEDY

1. Add 1 tablespoon of dried dandelion root and 1 tablespoon of dried milk thistle to a cup of hot water and let it steep for 15 minutes.
2. After 15 minutes, strain the water into another cup using a fine mesh strainer and drink it.
3. Drink this remedy up to 4 times per day to treat your fibroids.

TIPS:

- Adopting a healthy diet and learning to eat the right foods is an important part of the process to treat fibroids. Processed foods, fatty foods and sugars should be replaced with organic produce such as vegetables, beans, seeds and nuts.

- Living with fibroids can be miserable if you suffer from many of the uncomfortable symptoms. But there is no need to suffer in silence as fibroids can be dealt with and in most cases treatment can be minimal.

- With more and more studies proving that a hysterectomy is perhaps not the only solution or even the answer to a severe case of fibroids, there is now a lot more information available on the various methods currently used in the prevention and treatment of fibroids. The condition itself is now widely recognized and is taken a lot more seriously.

Women, if you've not already done so; put your mind at ease, talk with your Gynecologist about the many options to treat Fibroids.

FLU

NATURAL HOME REMEDY

GINGER, MANUKA HONEY & LEMON JUICE

HOW THE REMEDY WORKS

Flu (also known as influenza) is a contagious viral infection that affects the upper respiratory system. Its symptoms include congestion, fever, headaches, pain throughout the body and weakness. When you feel the very first stages of a cold or flu, try drinking some of this tea remedy several times a day.

This ginger, honey and lemon remedy treats flu in the following ways:

1. **Ginger:** Ginger reduces the congestion associated with flu and directly combats the influenza virus.
2. **Manuka Honey:** Manuka honey treats the influenza virus and soothes many of the associated symptoms.
3. **Lemon Juice:** Lemon juice's antiviral properties make it very effective at fighting the influenza virus while its high vitamin C content strengthens your immune system.

HOW TO PREPARE THE REMEDY

1. Add 1 tablespoon of lemon juice, 1 teaspoon of ground ginger and 1 teaspoon of manuka honey to a cup of hot water, let it steep for 5 minutes and drink it.
2. Use this remedy up to 4 times per day until the flu subsides.

TIP:

You can even drink this tea remedy as a preventative if you think you may have been exposed to any viruses.

FRIZZY HAIR

NATURAL HOME REMEDY

AVOCADO & MANUKA HONEY

HOW THE REMEDY WORKS

Frizzy hair occurs when your hair lacks moisture and can lead to dull, dry, unmanageable hair.

This avocado and manuka honey remedy helps to treat frizzy hair in the following ways:

1. **Avocado:** The healthy fats and vitamin E in avocado are very beneficial to the hair and help to lock in moisture and make it more manageable.

2. **Manuka Honey:** Honey has a hydrating effect on the hair and also gives it a vibrant shine.

HOW TO PREPARE THE REMEDY

1. Warm 2 tablespoons of honey in a saucepan and combine it with a mashed avocado.
2. Massage the mixture into your scalp thoroughly, and then wrap your hair in a towel for 30 minutes.
3. After 30 minutes, remove the towel, comb your hair thoroughly and then wash it.
4. Use this remedy 3 times per week until the frizzy hair subsides.

TIP:

Water is a great solution for fizzy hair: Avoid brushing dry hair, instead comb your dry hair with wet fingers. Remember not to over process your hair with relaxers and straighteners; they will make your hair dry and brittle (frizzy).

Avocado & Manuka Honey is a great hair conditioner. Make sure you always have on hand!

Also See Remedy For Dry Scalp In Part 1

GALLSTONES

NATURAL HOME REMEDY

APPLE CIDER VINEGAR & PEPPERMINT

HOW THE REMEDY WORKS

Gallstones are hard, crystalline deposits that build up in the gallbladder. They can cause severe pain, bloating and digestive problems. Gallstone attacks usually happen after you eat. Signs of a gallstone attack may include nausea, vomiting, or pain in the abdomen, back, or just under the right arm. The two types of gallstones are cholesterol and pigment stones: **Cholesterol stones**, usually yellow-green in color, consist primarily of hardened cholesterol. According to niddk.nih.gov, in the United States, more than 80 percent of gallstones are cholesterol stones. **Pigment stones**, dark in color, are made of bilirubin (a brownish yellow substance found in bile).

This apple cider vinegar and peppermint remedy helps to treat gallstones in the following ways:

1. **Apple Cider Vinegar:** Apple cider vinegar helps to regulate cholesterol levels in the body (cholesterol is a key cause of gallstones) and also dissolves gallstones.
2. **Peppermint:** Peppermint supports healthy digestion and soothes gallbladder pain.

HOW TO PREPARE THE REMEDY

1. Add 1 tablespoon of apple cider vinegar and 1 tablespoon of dried peppermint to a cup of hot water and let it steep for 5 minutes.
2. After 5 minutes, strain the water into another cup using a fine mesh strainer and drink it.
3. Drink this remedy up to 4 times per day until the gallstones disappear.

TIPS:

According to research diets high in calories and refined carbohydrates and low in fiber increase the risk of gallstones. Refined carbohydrates are grains processed to remove bran and germ, which contain nutrients and fiber. Examples of refined carbohydrates include white bread and white rice.

Good news - You can decrease your risk of gallstones by maintaining a healthy weight through proper diet and nutrition.

GAS

NATURAL HOME REMEDY

BAKING SODA & CINNAMON

HOW THE REMEDY WORKS

Gas is air in the digestive tract—the large, muscular tube that extends from the mouth to the anus. Gas leaves the body when you burp through the mouth or pass gas through the anus. Gas in the digestive tract is usually caused by swallowing air and the breakdown of certain foods in the large intestine. Everyone pass gas, and according to studies passing gas around 13 to 21 times a day is normal. However, many people think they burp or pass gas too often and that they have too much gas. Excess gas can be embarrassing and also lead to abdominal bloating, abdominal pain and uncontrollable flatulence.

This baking soda and cinnamon remedy helps to treat gas in the following ways:

1. **Baking Soda:** Baking soda is an effective antacid that releases gas from the stomach.
2. **Cinnamon:** Cinnamon calms the stomach and helps to protect against the buildup of gas.

HOW TO PREPARE THE REMEDY

1. Add 1 teaspoon of baking soda and 1 teaspoon of ground cinnamon to a glass of cold water mix it well and drink it.
2. Drink this remedy up to 4 times per day until the gas subsides.

TIPS:

Eating habits and diet affect the amount of gas you have:
Eating and drinking too fast can cause you to swallow more air.
You may have more gas after you eat certain carbohydrates – a few examples:

- Beans
- Vegetables such as broccoli, cauliflower, cabbage, brussels sprouts, onions, mushrooms, artichokes, and asparagus
- Fruits such as pears, apples, and peaches
- Whole grains such as whole wheat and bran
- Milk and milk products such as cheese, ice cream, and yogurt

Swallowing less air and changing what you eat can help prevent or reduce gas. Try the following:

- Eat more slowly
- If you smoke, quit
- Don't chew gum or suck on hard candies
- Avoid carbonated drinks, such as soda and beer
- If you wear dentures - make sure they fit correctly

Remember - Foods that cause gas for one person may not cause gas for someone else.

GUM DISEASE

NATURAL HOME REMEDY

ALOE VERA & SEA SALT

HOW THE REMEDY WORKS

Gum disease (also known as gingivitis/periodontal disease) most commonly, develops when plaque is allowed to build up along and under the gum line. Gum disease can cause bleeding, red or swollen gums, bad breath and even tooth loss. Gingivitis is a mild form of gum disease with inflammation of the gum. Gingivitis is usually very mild and many people may have it and not know. This form of gum disease does not include any loss of bone and tissue that hold teeth in place. When gingivitis is not treated, it can advance to periodontitis (which means - inflammation around the tooth). In periodontitis, gums pull away from the teeth and form spaces (called - pockets) that become infected. Periodontal diseases range from simple gum inflammation to serious disease that may result in major damage to the soft tissue and bone that support the teeth. In the worst cases, teeth are lost.

This aloe vera and sea salt remedy helps to treat gum disease in the following ways:

1. **Aloe Vera**: Aloe Vera is a natural anti-inflammatory and can soothe many of the painful symptoms of gum disease.
2. **Sea Salt:** Sea salt is packed with minerals that fight many of the infections that cause gum disease.

HOW TO PREPARE THE REMEDY

1. Massage a teaspoon of aloe vera gel into your gums and leave it for 30 minutes.
2. After 30 minutes, add 1 teaspoon of sea salt to a cup of warm water, mix it well until the sea salt is fully dissolved, swirl the solution around your mouth for 30 seconds and then spit it out.
3. Use this remedy up to 4 times per day until the gum disease subsides.

TIP:

The main goal of treatment is to control gum infection. It is important to keep up good daily care of teeth and gum. If you smoke consider quitting.

HEADACHES

NATURAL HOME REMEDY

LAVENDER OIL & ROSEMARY OIL

HOW THE REMEDY WORKS

Headaches are something that many people experience at some point in their lives and can be caused by a variety of factors. Some common triggers are smoking, hunger or skipping meals, certain foods, depression, bad sleeping habits, head injury, loud music, long car rides, overexertion, strong odors, common colds, menstruation, stress, and caffeine.

This lavender oil and rosemary oil remedy helps to treat headaches in the following ways:

1. **Lavender Oil:** Lavender oil has a soothing effect on the body and mind and can make headaches melt away.
2. **Rosemary Oil:** Rosemary oil is a potent anti-inflammatory that can ease many of the symptoms associated with headaches.

HOW TO PREPARE THE REMEDY

1. Massage 2 drops of lavender oil and 2 drops of rosemary oil into your forehead.
2. Use this remedy up to 4 times per day until the headache subsides.

TIP:

Not all headaches are serious, but they can be. Check with your doctor if you have persistent headaches to rule out any serious health problems.

HEARTBURN

NATURAL HOME REMEDY

PEPPERMINT & SLIPPERY ELM

HOW THE REMEDY WORKS

Heartburn is a disorder that causes discomfort and a burning sensation in the chest. The production of stomach acids increase when a person is stressed, which can cause heartburn to become worse. Take a few deep breaths, breathing in through the nose and out through the mouth and try to relax. Foods that are known to cause heartburn should be avoided. Even though the specific foods that cause one person to suffer from heartburn do not mean it is going to bother another person. A few of the common food products that cause heartburn include foods that are spicy, orange juice, mint, chocolate, vinegar, greasy foods, tomato sauce, and garlic.

This peppermint and slippery elm remedy treats heartburn in the following ways:

1. **Peppermint**: Peppermint helps to reduce indigestion (one of the leading causes of heartburn).
2. **Slippery Elm:** Slippery elm protects your esophagus against the acids that cause heartburn.

HOW TO PREPARE THE REMEDY

1. Add 1 tablespoon of dried peppermint and 1 teaspoon of ground slippery elm to a cup of hot water and let it steep for 5 minutes.
2. After 5 minutes, strain the water into another cup using a fine mesh strainer and drink it.
3. Drink this remedy up to 4 times per day until the heartburn subsides.

TIPS:

1. **Eat slowly** Eating much too fast can trigger the occurrence of heartburn. Eating slower is not only healthier for you but it can help prevent problems with heartburn.
2. **Don't exercise on a full stomach** The process of digestion actually slows down when a person engages in a vigorous workout. Wait at least a couple of hours after mealtime before you engage in strenuous activities or exercise routines.
3. **Stay in an upright position after meals** When you remain in an upright position after you have eaten a meal, it decreases the chances of stomach acids coming back up and making their way into the esophagus.

HIGH BLOOD PRESSURE

NATURAL HOME REMEDY

CAYENNE & LEMON JUICE

HOW THE REMEDY WORKS

High blood pressure (also known as hypertension) is a serious health disorder. Even though it typically has no symptoms, high blood pressure can have deadly health consequences if not treated. Blood pressure is the force of blood against the walls of your arteries. Your blood pressure is always rising and falling throughout the day and if it rises and stays that way over time, you have high blood pressure. When you have high blood pressure it puts more pressure on the heart, making it work harder than usual. Anyone can have high blood pressure. According to the American Heart Association about 80 million American adults have been diagnosed with high blood pressure.

Even though these home remedies are all natural, that doesn't mean that you still can't have a potentially dangerous interaction with your other medications. Be Safe: As stated above - High blood pressure can be a serious health problem. If you are under a doctor's care and taking prescription medications, talk to your doctor before you try any self treatment.

This cayenne and lemon juice remedy treats high blood pressure in the following ways:

1. **Cayenne:** Cayenne regulates blood pressure and promotes healthy blood flow in your body.
2. **Lemon Juice**: The antioxidants in lemon juice protect and repair your blood vessels from the damage caused by high blood pressure.

HOW TO PREPARE THE REMEDY

1. Add 1 tablespoon of lemon juice and ½ teaspoon of cayenne powder to a cup of hot water, mix well and drink it.
2. Drink this remedy up to 4 times per day to treat high blood pressure.

REMEDY VARIATIONS:

1. **Use fresh lemon juice:** About half a lemon, and add to an 8 ounce glass of water. Drink throughout your day, two to three hours apart.
2. **Eating fresh papaya daily**: on an empty stomach, has been shown in some people to help lower blood pressure.
3. **Garlic**: This may be one of the best known remedies for treating high blood pressure. You can easily add it to many of the foods you prepare, about 1 clove per day.
4. **Exercise:** If you are not already doing this, get active. It may take as little as thirty minutes a day of physical activity or exercise to control your blood pressure and better your health.

HOT FLASHES

NATURAL HOME REMEDY

RED CLOVER & SAGE

HOW THE REMEDY WORKS

Hot flashes are a condition that often affect women going through menopause and cause them to suddenly experience intense heat in their body. Hot flashes are one of the most common symptom complaints from menopause sufferers.

This red clover and sage remedy helps to treat hot flashes in the following ways:

1. **Red Clover:** Red clover helps to regulate the hormones that cause hot flashes.
2. **Sage:** Sage naturally combats the symptoms of hot flashes.

HOW TO PREPARE THE REMEDY

1. Add 1 teaspoon of dried red clover and 1 teaspoon of dried sage to a cup of hot water and let it steep for 5 minutes.

2. After 5 minutes, strain the water into another cup using a fine mesh strainer and drink it.
3. Drink this remedy up to 4 times per day to combat hot flashes.

TIPS:

There are also lifestyle changes you can try to help reduce hot flashes:

- **Exercise** can improve your quality of life and may help with hot flashes.
- Dress in layers, and remove as needed at the start of a hot flash.
- Have a drink of cold water when you feel a hot flash coming on.

HYPOTHYROIDISM

NATURAL HOME REMEDY

COCONUT OIL & GINGER

HOW THE REMEDY WORKS

Hypothyroidism is a common disorder in which the thyroid gland doesn't produce enough thyroid hormone (also called - underactive thyroid).The thyroid gland is located in the front lower part of your neck. Hormones released by the thyroid gland travel through your bloodstream and affect nearly every part of your body, from your heart and brain, to your muscles and skin. The thyroid controls how your body's cells use energy from food, a process called metabolism. Among other things, your metabolism affects your body's temperature, your heartbeat, and how well you burn calories. If you don't have enough thyroid hormone, your body processes slow down. That means your body makes less energy, and your metabolism becomes sluggish.

Some common symptoms of hypothyroidism include: fatigue, increased sensitivity to cold, constipation, dry skin, muscle cramping, weight gain, depression and brittle fingernails and hair. Fortunately, there are natural remedies that can help control this health problem. Also consult with your healthcare provider for proper diagnosis and treatment of this condition. Use home remedies as an add-on treatment.

This coconut oil and ginger remedy helps to treat hypothyroidism in the following ways:

1. **Coconut Oil:** The healthy fats in coconut oil support your thyroid and enhance your metabolism.
2. **Ginger:** Ginger contains a range of nutrients that boost your thyroid and help it function properly.

HOW TO PREPARE THE REMEDY

1. Add 1 tablespoon of coconut oil and 1 teaspoon of ground ginger to a cup of hot water, let it steep for 5 minutes and drink it.
2. Drink this remedy up to 4 times per day to treat hypothyroidism.

REMEDY VARIATION:

Apple cider vinegar may also help with thyroid disorder. It is believed that it helps detoxification, restores acid alkaline balance, and helps regulate hormones and improve energy metabolism.

- Add two tablespoons of organic apple cider vinegar to a glass of warm water.
- Mix in a little raw or manuka honey.
- Drink this remedy daily on a regular basis to treat hypothyroidism.

INDIGESTION

NATURAL HOME REMEDY

GINGER

HOW THE REMEDY WORKS

Ginger has a long history as a natural remedy in Asian, Arabic and Indian cultures with the Chinese using ginger as a natural remedy for indigestion for over 2000 years. Studies into ginger have shown that it is a carminative (a substance that helps to eliminate intestinal gas from the body) and intestinal spasmolytic (a substance that calms and relaxes the intestinal tract). It's also an anti-inflammatory which helps to prevent inflammation in the stomach and relieve any painful associated symptoms.

HOW TO PREPARE THE REMEDY

Ginger can be consumed in a number of different ways but one of the simplest solutions is ginger tea. To prepare ginger tea, follow the instructions below:

1. Add 1 teaspoon of ground ginger to 1 cup of boiling water.

2. Mix the ground ginger and boiling water together thoroughly, let the ground ginger steep for 5 minutes and drink it.

TIP:

For the best results with this ginger root tea indigestion remedy, drink it up to 4 times per day. It's important that you drink no more than 4 cups of ginger tea each day as too much ginger can actually aggravate your digestive system and cause further digestive problems.

REMEDY VARIATIONS:

To calm your stomach at an even faster rate, try mixing ginger with the following natural indigestion remedies:

1. **Coriander:** Coriander contains the oils borneol and linalool which are powerful anti-inflammatories that promote proper digestion. To combat indigestion with coriander and ginger tea, add 1 teaspoon of ground coriander and 1 teaspoon of ground ginger to 1 cup of boiling water, let it steep for 5 minutes and then drink it.
2. **Fennel Seeds:** Fennel seeds are packed with oils that support the digestive system and treat indigestion. To combat indigestion with fennel seeds and ginger tea, add 1 teaspoon of ground fennel seeds and 1 teaspoon of ground ginger to 1 cup of boiling water, let it steep for 5 minutes and then drink it.

3. **Mint Tea:** Mint tea has a calming effect on your stomach and helps to prevent digestive complications. To combat indigestion with mint tea and ginger, add 1 mint teabag and 1 teaspoon of ground ginger to 1 cup of boiling water, let it steep for 5 minutes, then remove the teabag and drink it.
4. **Orange Juice:** Orange juice is loaded with ascorbic acid and citric acid which enhance your digestive capacity and reduce your risk of digestive problems.
5. To combat indigestion with orange juice and ginger, add 1 teaspoon of ground ginger to 1 glass of orange juice, mix it well and drink it.

INFLAMMATION

NATURAL HOME REMEDY

CAT' S CLAW & GREEN TEA

HOW THE REMEDY WORKS

Inflammation can affect any part of the body and is usually characterized by swelling, redness and pain. Swelling (inflammation) is the body's natural reaction to an injury. Inflammation can happen anywhere on the skin, within the body, and even inside the arteries. Chronic inflammation is silent. Scientists are now learning inflammation may play a part in many of the diseases that come with aging, including coronary artery disease. Fortunately, you can help control inflammation.

This cat's claw and green tea remedy helps to treat inflammation in the following ways:

1. **Cat's Claw:** Cat's claw blocks many of the substances that cause inflammation in the body.
2. **Green Tea:** Green tea is packed with powerful and natural anti-inflammatory.

HOW TO PREPARE THE REMEDY

1. Crush 1 teaspoon of dry green tea leaves and 1 teaspoon of ground cat's claw using a mortar and pestle.
2. Mix these crushed ingredients with a small amount of water to form a paste.
3. Apply the paste to the inflamed part of the body for 10 minutes and then wash it clean with warm water.
4. Use this remedy every couple of hours until the inflammation subsides.

FOOD REMEDIES:

NATURE'S OWN ANTI-INFLAMMATORY:

1. **Oil:** Extra virgin Olive Oil, Grape Seed, and Avocado Oils, keeping inflammation down.
2. **Fish:** Salmon, Snapper, Cod, Halibut and bass are all high in omega-3 fatty acid.
3. **Nuts:** Walnuts, almonds, sunflower seeds and flax seeds - Just two tablespoons of ground flaxseed contain more than 140 percent daily value of the inflammation-reducing omega-3 fatty acids.
4. **Dark Chocolate:** At least 70% cocoa, (no milk chocolate) a delicious way to keep inflammation down.

INSOMNIA

NATURAL HOME REMEDY

MILK & NUTMEG

HOW THE REMEDY WORKS

Insomnia is a sleep disorder which makes it difficult or impossible to fall asleep, hard to stay asleep or both. Insomnia is a common problem that takes a toll on your energy, mood, health, and ability to function during the day. Insomnia symptoms may include:

- Difficulty falling asleep at night
- Awakening during the night
- Awakening too early
- Not feeling well rested after a night's sleep
- Daytime tiredness or sleepiness
- Irritability, depression or anxiety

This milk and nutmeg remedy helps to treat insomnia in the following ways:

1. **Milk:** Milk contains a range of amino acids that stimulate sleep.
2. **Nutmeg:** Nutmeg is a natural sedative and makes falling asleep easier.

HOW TO PREPARE THE REMEDY

1. Add ½ teaspoon of nutmeg powder to a glass of warm milk and drink it 30 minutes before you sleep.
2. Drink this remedy nightly to treat insomnia.

TIPS:

Chronic insomnia can contribute to serious health problems. Talk with your healthcare provider if you suffer from chronic insomnia.

Insomnia is often categorized by how long it lasts:

1. **Transient:** insomnia lasts for a few days.
2. **Short-term:** insomnia lasts for no more than 3 weeks.
3. **Chronic insomnia:** occurs at least 3 nights per week for 1 month or longer.

Source: Insomnia | University of Maryland Medical Center
http://umm.edu/health/medical/reports/articles/insomnia

IRRITABLE BOWEL SYNDROME

NATURAL HOME REMEDY

FLAX SEEDS & YOGURT

HOW THE REMEDY WORKS

Irritable bowel syndrome (also known as IBS) is a gastrointestinal disorder that can cause constipation, diarrhea and stomach pain. IBS is one of the most common disorders that doctors report. Studies estimate that irritable bowel syndrome affects 10 to 15 percent of U.S. adults. According to the National Institute of Diabetes and Digestive and Kidney Diseases (NIH) people with IBS may have diarrhea, constipation, or both. Some people with IBS have only diarrhea or only constipation. Some people have symptoms of both or have diarrhea sometimes and constipation other times. People often have symptoms soon after eating a meal. Other symptoms of IBS are:

- Bloating
- The feeling that you haven't finished a bowel movement
- Whitish mucus in your stool

Women with IBS often have more symptoms during their menstrual periods.

This flax seeds and yogurt remedy helps to treat IBS in the following ways:

1. **Flax Seeds:** Flax seeds are rich in fiber and healthy fats which promote good digestive health and soothe your bowel.
2. **Yogurt:** Yogurt helps to remove harmful bacteria from your bowel and alleviate many of the unpleasant symptoms of IBS.

HOW TO PREPARE THE REMEDY

1. Sprinkle 1 tablespoon of flax seeds into 1 cup of yogurt and eat it.
2. Use this remedy up to 2 times per day to treat IBS.

REMEDY VARIATION:

Peppermint Oil: Peppermint is a natural antispasmodic that relaxes smooth muscles in the intestines. The preferred form of peppermint is enteric-coated capsules. They break down in the intestines, not in the stomach, where they could cause heartburn. Take 1-2 capsules (each containing 0.2 ml of peppermint oil), two or three times a day, preferably between meals.

ITCHING

NATURAL HOME REMEDY

BASIL & PEPPERMINT

HOW THE REMEDY WORKS

Itching is a common sensation on the skin that can affect anyone and ranges from mild to severe. Itching is irritating and makes you want to scratch to relieve the feeling. Some symptoms of itching may be associated with: dry skin, rashes such as poison ivy, insect bites and irritation from clothes. Itching can be diffuse (generalized all over the body) or localized, all over or confined to a specific spot.

This basil and peppermint remedy helps to treat itching in the following ways:

1. **Basil:** Basil contains a range of compounds that reduce itching.
2. **Dried Peppermint:** Peppermint has a cooling effect on the skin and can soothe the sensations of itching.

HOW TO PREPARE THE REMEDY

1. Crush 1 teaspoon of basil and 1 teaspoon of dried peppermint using a mortar and pestle.
2. Mix these crushed ingredients with a small amount of water to form a paste.
3. Gently scrub the paste into the itchy area for 2 minutes and then wash it clean with warm water.
4. Use this remedy every time you start to feel an itch.

TIPS:

Things you can do to help avoid itching:

- Wear loose fitting, 100% cotton clothing.
- Avoid skin irritants, such as wool, pet hair, harsh soaps, and perfumed lotions.
- Apply a cool compress to itchy areas. A cool washcloth may be enough to relieve itching.

Remember: You should never ignore itching, if you have severe or chronic itching, check with your healthcare provider.

JAW PAIN

NATURAL HOME REMEDY

GINGER & ST JOHN'   S WORT

HOW THE REMEDY WORKS

Jaw pain is any kind of pain or discomfort in the jaw area, which includes the lower jaw. Jaw pain can be caused by fractures, grinding of the teeth and poor jaw alignment. Jaw pain may be triggered by various activities, such as eating, swallowing or merely habitually chewing gum.

This ginger and St John's wort remedy helps to relieve jaw pain in the following ways:

1. **Ginger:** Ginger reduces the pain, redness and swelling associated with jaw pain and allows your jaw to move more freely.
2. **St John's Wort:** St John's wort soothes the muscles in your jaw and allows you to recover from jaw pain quickly.

HOW TO PREPARE THE REMEDY

1. Crush 1 teaspoon of ground ginger and 1 teaspoon of ground St John's wort using a mortar and pestle.
2. Mix these crushed ingredients with a small amount of water to form a paste.
3. Apply the paste to the painful area of the jaw for 10 minutes and then wash it clean with warm water.
4. Use this remedy every couple of hours until the jaw pain subsides.

TIPS:

Below are some great tips to help relieve jaw pain:

1. Moist heat - Moist heat from a heat pack or a hot water bottle wrapped in a warm, moist towel can improve function and reduce pain. Be careful to avoid burning yourself when using heat.
2. Ice - Ice packs can decrease inflammation and also numb pain and promote healing. Do not place an ice pack directly on your skin. Keep the pack wrapped in a clean cloth while you are using it. Do not use an ice pack for more than 10 - 15 minutes.

Remember to avoid hard, crunchy, and chewy foods. Allow your jaw pain to heal before stretching your mouth to eat foods such as, corn on the cob, apples, or whole fruits.

JET LAG

NATURAL HOME REMEDY

GINGER & LEMON JUICE

HOW THE REMEDY WORKS

Jet lag is a temporary disorder that causes fatigue (extreme tiredness) and insomnia experienced by people who travel across multiple time zones by plane. A jet lag sufferer may also experience anxiety, constipation, diarrhea, nausea and dehydration. Jet lag is also defined as the feeling similar to symptoms such as fatigue, insomnia, and general irritability caused by a tired mind.

This ginger and lemon juice remedy helps to treat jet lag in the following ways:

1. **Ginger:** Ginger helps your body to reset and relax when switching between time zones.
2. **Lemon Juice:** Lemon juice helps to maintain healthy digestion while you fly and also keeps you hydrated.

HOW TO PREPARE THE REMEDY

1. Add 1 tablespoon of lemon juice and 1 teaspoon of ground ginger to a travel mug.
2. Once on board, ask a flight attendant to fill the travel mug with hot water, let it steep for 5 minutes and then drink it.
3. Drink this remedy up to 4 times during your flight to avoid jet lag.

TIPS:

- Stay hydrated.
- Drink water before, during, and after your flight to counteract dehydration.
- It is advisable to drink constantly throughout the flight with clear water to keep the body hydrated and supplied. As dehydration sets in, the flow of blood is slowed down.
- Avoid alcohol or caffeine a few hours before you plan to sleep. Alcohol and caffeine can disrupt sleep and may cause dehydration.

JOINT PAIN

NATURAL HOME REMEDY

NETTLE LEAF & TURMERIC

HOW THE REMEDY WORKS

Joint pain can occur in the ankles, hips, knees, wrists, fingers, shoulders and toes. Joint pain is extremely common and can affect any part of your body. It may be linked to arthritis, bursitis, and muscle pain. No matter what causes it, joint pain can be very bothersome. Joint pain can range from mildly irritating to debilitating. It may go away after a few weeks (acute), or last for several weeks or months (chronic). Even short-term pain and swelling in the joints can affect your quality of life. Whatever the cause of joint pain, you can usually manage it. For an alternative treatment try the natural remedy below.

This nettle leaf and turmeric remedy helps to treat joint pain in the following ways:

1. **Nettle Leaf:** Nettle leaf has a soothing effect on your joints and naturally relieves pain.
2. **Turmeric:** Turmeric protects against inflammation in the joints and can reduce any pain, redness and swelling.

HOW TO PREPARE THE REMEDY

1. Add 1 tablespoon of dried nettle leaf and 1 teaspoon of turmeric to a cup of hot water and let it steep for 5 minutes.
2. After 5 minutes, strain the water into another cup using a fine mesh strainer and drink it.
3. Drink this remedy up to 4 times per day until the joint pain subsides.

TIPS:

For non arthritis joint pain, both rest and exercise are important. Warm baths, massage, and stretching exercises should be used as often as possible.

PART 3: K THRU P

"A wise man should consider that health is the greatest of human blessings, and learn how by his own thought to derive benefit from his illnesses."

— Hippocrates

KIDNEY STONES

NATURAL HOME REMEDY

Apple Cider Vinegar, Watermelon & Wheatgrass Juice

HOW THE REMEDY WORKS

Kidney stones are hard, insoluble calcium compounds that form in the kidneys and can lead to pain and frequent urination. Kidney stones form when the urine becomes concentrated, allowing minerals to crystallize and stick together.

This apple cider vinegar, watermelon and wheatgrass juice remedy treats kidney stones in the following ways:

1. **Apple Cider Vinegar:** Apple cider vinegar dissolves kidney stones and reduces the pain that they cause.
2. **Watermelon:** Watermelon boosts your kidneys and helps them to deal with kidney stones more efficiently.
3. **Wheatgrass Juice:** Wheatgrass juice contains a range of nutrients that naturally treat kidney stones.

HOW TO PREPARE THE REMEDY

1. Blend 1 cup of watermelon, 1 cup of wheatgrass juice and 1 tablespoon of apple cider vinegar in a blender until smooth and then drink it.
2. Drink this remedy up to 4 times per day until the kidney stones disappear.

TIPS: Drink More Water

- According to medical evidence, problems with crystals forming into kidney stones will worsen when a person does not drink enough fluids.

- Eat some parsley with your meals. Parsley tracks all the way back to Hippocrates who used it for medicinal purposes, for cure alls and as an antidote for poisons. He also used it for ridding kidney and bladder stones. Many of these prior claims have been validated through modern science and it is true that Parsley is rich in vitamin A and C and is also shown to clear toxins from the body and reduces inflammation. Parsley has three times the amount of Vitamin C than oranges.

LICE

NATURAL HOME REMEDY

EXTRA VIRGIN OLIVE OIL & WHITE VINEGAR

HOW THE REMEDY WORKS

Lice (also known as head lice) are small parasites that feed on blood from the scalp. An infestation of head lice, called pediculosis capitis, most often affects children and usually results from the direct transfer of lice from the hair of one person to the hair of another.

TIP: HOW TO AVOID HEAD LICE:

- Do not share combs or brushes
- Do not share hats
- Be vigilant for head lice - especially after sleepovers
- Remember, head lice do not jump or fly

Head lice don't carry bacterial or viral infectious diseases. Good news you can get rid of them! They can be treated with natural home remedies.

Try this - extra virgin olive oil and white vinegar remedy to treats head lice in the following ways:

1. **Extra Virgin Olive Oil:** Extra virgin olive oil smothers and suffocates lice.
2. **White Vinegar:** White vinegar loosens lice eggs and clears them out of your hair.

HOW TO PREPARE THE REMEDY

1. Warm ½ cup of extra virgin olive oil and 1 tablespoon of white vinegar in a saucepan and mix it well.
2. Massage the mixture into your scalp thoroughly, and then wrap your hair in a towel for 30 minutes.
3. After 30 minutes, remove the towel, comb your hair thoroughly and then wash it.
4. Use this remedy daily until the lice disappear.

MENOPAUSE

NATURAL HOME REMEDY

CHASTEBERRY & CINNAMON

HOW THE REMEDY WORKS

Menopause is the natural ceasing of fertility and menstruation in women. While it is a natural part of any woman's life, it often causes a range of unpleasant symptoms including breast pain, hot flashes, thinning hair and tiredness.

This chasteberry and cinnamon remedy helps to soothe these symptoms in the following ways:

1. **Chasteberry:** Chasteberry helps to balance hormone levels in menopausal women.
2. **Cinnamon:** Cinnamon can ease and reduce the pain caused by menopause.

HOW TO PREPARE THE REMEDY

1. Add 1 teaspoon of chasteberry powder and 1 teaspoon of ground cinnamon to a cup of hot water, mix it well and let it steep for 5 minutes.
2. After 5 minutes, strain the water into another cup using a fine mesh strainer and drink it.
3. Drink this remedy up to 4 times per day to ease the symptoms of menopause

TIP:

Beetroot juice is effective in providing those suffering from menopause with relief. This natural remedy for menopause has been proven successful on a number of occasions. Beetroot juice contains all the necessary nutrients that help alleviate menopausal disturbances. Beetroot can be eaten in a salad, juice (use vegetable juicer - 8 oz. daily), or boiled with the peel on, make sure to remove peel before eating.

MENSTRUAL CRAMPS

NATURAL HOME REMEDY

BASIL & FENNEL SEEDS

HOW THE REMEDY WORKS

Menstrual cramps are painful muscle spasms that occur during the menstrual cycle. Some women may experience intense pain in the lower abdomen, back and thighs. Some women may also have headaches, nausea, dizziness or fainting, diarrhea or constipation.

This basil and fennel seeds remedy helps to soothe menstrual cramps in the following ways:

1. **Basil:** Basil is a natural analgesic and can help to reduce the pain associated with menstrual cramps.
2. **Fennel Seeds**: Fennel seeds relax the uterine muscles and this helps to relieve any cramping.

HOW TO PREPARE THE REMEDY

1. Add 1 teaspoon of ground basil and 1 teaspoon of ground fennel seeds to a cup of boiling water, let it steep for 5 minutes and drink it.
2. Drink this remedy up to 4 times per day to soothe menstrual cramps.

REMEDY VARIATION/TIP:

1. **Herbal Teas:** Chamomile, Mint, Raspberry and Blackberry can help soothe tense muscles. Prepare same as above or use tea bags.
2. **Exercise:** Regular workouts will also help decrease the severity of cramps.

MIGRAINES

NATURAL HOME REMEDY

EUCALYPTUS OIL & PEPPERMINT OIL

HOW THE REMEDY WORKS

Migraines are a severe form of headache that can also cause blind spots, flashes of light in your vision and tingling in your limbs. It is very important that you learn how to prevent a headache. You will find that there are many triggers and dangers to headaches. You will find that it may take a whole new way to life to get the headaches to stop. It is very important that you consider the following information; that you go to see a doctor for your persistent headaches, your doctor will be able to rule out some things. Things like stress and depression can play a huge part in your headaches. You not only need to learn how to be healthy, but you have to feel healthy.

This eucalyptus oil and peppermint oil remedy helps to treat migraines in the following ways:

1. **Eucalyptus Oil:** Eucalyptus oil helps to relieve the tension associated with migraines.

2. **Peppermint Oil:** Peppermint oil is a natural pain reliever and reduces many of the unpleasant symptoms of migraines.

HOW TO PREPARE THE REMEDY

1. Massage 2 drops of eucalyptus oil and 2 drops of peppermint oil into your forehead.
2. Use this remedy up to 4 times per day until the migraine subsides.

TIPS:

- Stay hydrated: Dehydration can also play a part in your headaches. Water is key to reducing the average time frame of a headache or a migraine. As with a healthy diet, the regular consumption of water can help to prevent the onset of headaches and migraines. In addition to drinking plain water, another home and natural remedy for headaches and migraines that comes recommended is honey. Many headache and migraine sufferers report a decrease or complete elimination in pain when drinking a glass of water with a teaspoon of honey.

- A cold compress can also and should be used to help treat a migraine or a headache. A zip lock bag filled with ice or a cold washcloth can be used. Although a cold compress is an ideal way to seek relief from a headache or a migraine, there are also individuals who claim that heat provides them with assistance. If you would like to try this approach, start with warm washcloths or towels around the neck and armpits. Those suffering from migraines are encouraged to limit their exposure to household lights, sunlight, television, and computer screens.

Also See Headache Remedies In Part 2

MORNING SICKNESS

NATURAL HOME REMEDY

GINGER, LEMON JUICE & PEPPERMINT

HOW THE REMEDY WORKS

More than 50% of all pregnant women experience morning sickness according to the American Pregnancy Association. Morning sickness is very common. Most pregnant women have at least some nausea. The exact cause of morning sickness is unknown. Morning sickness is a type of nausea, vomiting, or both; experienced by many women in the early stages of pregnancy. Morning sickness usually occurs during the morning however, it can occur at anytime of the day. For some women morning sickness lingers throughout their pregnancy.

This ginger, lemon and peppermint remedy helps to treat morning sickness in the following ways:

1. **Ginger:** Ginger helps to protect against nausea and vomiting.
2. **Lemon Juice:** Lemon juice calms your stomach and soothes the symptoms of morning sickness.
3. **Peppermint:** Peppermint soothes your digestive tract and helps to keep morning sickness at bay.

HOW TO PREPARE THE REMEDY

1. Add 1 tablespoon of dried peppermint, 1 tablespoon of ground ginger and 1 teaspoon of lemon juice to a cup of hot water and let it steep for 5 minutes.
2. After 5 minutes, strain the water into another cup using a fine mesh strainer and drink it.
3. Drink this remedy up to 4 times per day to combat morning sickness.

TIPS:

Remember that morning sickness usually stops after the first 3 or 4 months of pregnancy. Keep a positive attitude and try the below tips:

- Drink fluids one half hour before or after a meal, but not with meals.
- Avoid eating spicy foods.
- Drink small amounts of fluids during the day to avoid dehydration.
- Get plenty of rest and nap during the day.
- Eat watermelon or yogurt to help fight morning sickness.

Also see Remedy for Nausea and Vomiting in Part 4

NASAL CONGESTION

NATURAL HOME REMEDY

LEMON OIL & LIME OIL

HOW THE REMEDY WORKS

Nasal congestion occurs when your nasal cavity becomes inflamed, swollen and full of mucus. A cold or allergies can cause membranes lining your nasal passages to become inflamed and irritated. They begin to produce excess mucus as a way of flushing out whatever is causing the irritation, such as an allergen.

This lemon oil and lime oil remedy helps to treat nasal congestion in the following ways:

1. **Lime Oil:** Lime oil fights many of the bacteria that contribute to nasal congestion.
2. **Tea Tree Oil:** Tea tree oil clears your nasal passages and reduces swelling.

HOW TO PREPARE THE REMEDY

1. Put 5 drops of lime oil and 5 drops of tea tree oil on a paper towel and then place it on your pillow while you sleep.
2. When you wake up, discard the paper towel, add 5 drops of lime oil and 5 drops of tea tree oil to a bowl of boiling water and breathe in the steam with deep breaths for 5 minutes.
3. Use this remedy up to 2 times per day until the nasal congestion is cleared.

TIPS:

- Drink plenty of clear fluids (water).
- Apply a warm, moist washcloth to your face several times a day.
- Remember, keeping your head elevated when lying down will help relieve nasal congestion.

NAUSEA

NATURAL HOME REMEDY

CLOVE & CUMIN SEEDS

HOW THE REMEDY WORKS

Nausea is a feeling of extreme sickness that often creates an urge to vomit. There are many causes of nausea; here are a few common causes:

- Emotional stress
- Food allergies
- Food poisoning
- Motion sickness
- Pregnancy
- Eating too much food
- Drinking too much alcohol

This clove and cumin seeds remedy helps to treat nausea in the following ways:

1. **Clove:** Clove's powerful natural aroma helps to overcome feelings of sickness and has a soothing effect on your stomach.
2. **Cumin Seeds:** Cumin seeds calm the digestive system which helps to reduce the occurrence of nausea.

HOW TO PREPARE THE REMEDY

1. Add 1 teaspoon of clove powder and 1 teaspoon of ground cumin seeds to a cup of hot water, let it steep for 5 minutes and drink it.
2. Drink this remedy up to 4 times per day to soothe nausea.

REMEDY VARIATION:

The best-researched use of ginger is in fighting nausea and vomiting, studies have shown that ginger is a versatile remedy. *Ginger* will help stop nausea.

Also See How To Prepare The Remedy for Morning Sickness in Part 3

More Benefits of Ginger - Anti-Inflammatory Healing Effects:

- It reduces pain and inflammation, making it valuable in managing arthritis, headaches, and menstrual cramps.
- It has a warming effect and stimulates circulation.
- It inhibits rhinovirus, which can cause the common cold.
- It inhibits such bacteria as Salmonella, which cause diarrhea.
- In the intestinal tract, it reduces gas and painful spasms.
- It may prevent stomach ulcers caused by non steroidal anti-inflammatory drugs, such as aspirin and ibuprofen.

TIPS: Try regularly spicing up your meals with fresh ginger.

- Add ginger and orange juice to puréed sweet potatoes.
- Add grated ginger to your baked apples.
- Spice up your healthy vegetables by adding freshly minced ginger.

NECK PAIN

NATURAL HOME REMEDY

ICE & LAVENDER OIL

HOW THE REMEDY WORKS

Neck pain is a common affliction that can be caused by poor posture, *sitting in an uncomfortable position and straining the neck. Also neck pain can come from common infections, such as virus infection of the throat. Neck pain is commonly associated with dull aching. Sometimes pain in the neck is worsened with movement of the neck or turning the head.

This ice and lavender oil remedy helps to treat neck pain in the following ways:

1. **Ice:** Ice soothes inflammation and reduces pain in the neck.
2. **Lavender Oil**: Lavender oil directly relieves neck pain and helps your neck muscles to relax.

HOW TO PREPARE THE REMEDY

1. Wrap 4 ice cubes in a small towel and hold it against your neck for 10 minutes.
2. After 10 minutes, massage 5 drops of lavender oil into your neck.
3. Use this remedy every couple of hours until the neck pain subsides.

TIPS:

- Try taking a bath with Epsom salts. Epsom salt is magnesium sulfate. It has a lot of medicinal qualities and can be absorbed into the skin easily.
- Avoid any activities that may be causing your neck pain, such as sitting for a long time at the computer.
- For more info on *Sitting Disease, visit **www.fitbodyandmore.com**

NERVE PAIN

NATURAL HOME REMEDY

CHAMOMILE OIL MARJORAM OIL & ST JOHN' S WORT OIL

HOW THE REMEDY WORKS

Nerve pain is often caused by damage to the nerves in your body but can also be the result of a pinched nerve. A pinched nerve can be caused by anything which increases pressure around a nerve. Common causes include body position such as leaning on elbows, habitually crossing legs, or poor posture.

This chamomile oil, marjoram oil and St John's wort oil remedy helps to treat nerve pain in the following ways:

1. **Chamomile Oil:** Chamomile oil has a soothing effect on your nerves and dulls any pain you may experience.
2. **Marjoram Oil:** Marjoram oil supports the nervous system and provides instant pain relief.
3. **St John's Wort Oil:** St John's wort oil is another natural pain reliever that can also help repair nerve damage.

HOW TO PREPARE THE REMEDY

1. Mix 1 tablespoon of St John's wort oil, 2 drops of chamomile oil and 2 drops of marjoram oil in a bowl and then massage this mixture directly into the painful nerves.
2. Use this remedy every couple of hours until the nerve pain subsides.

TIPS:

Check with your healthcare provider to make sure you are not deficient in B vitamins: The B vitamins are:

- B1 (thiamine)
- B2 (riboflavin)
- B3 (niacin)
- B5 (pantothenic acid)
- B6
- B7 (biotin)
- Folic acid
- These vitamins help the process your body uses to get or make energy from the food you eat. You can get B vitamins from proteins such as fish, poultry, meat, eggs, and dairy products; leafy green vegetables, beans, and peas.

- **B12** -Vitamin - B12's primary use by the body is aiding in the production of red blood cells, and in helping to maintain the health of the central nervous system. It keeps nerve cells healthy and protects against deterioration of the nerves.

NERVOUSNESS

NATURAL HOME REMEDY

ORANGE OIL & ROSEMARY OIL

HOW THE REMEDY WORKS

Nervousness is a common reaction to certain tasks and situations, being highly excitable; unnaturally or acutely uneasy or apprehensive. Nervousness is not considered a serious problem. Many people suffer from nervousness at some point or another, some even from irrational nervousness. However, when nervousness becomes overwhelming; never seems to go away, impacts your personal life, or is accompanied by severe physical symptoms, it's time to seek help.

This orange oil and rosemary oil remedy helps to treat nervousness in the following ways:

1. **Orange Oil:** Orange oil is uplifting, relaxing and helps keep nerves at bay.
2. **Rosemary Oil:** Rosemary oil naturally relaxes your body and mind.

HOW TO PREPARE THE REMEDY

1. Add 5 drops of orange oil and 5 drops of rosemary oil to a bowl of boiling water and breathe in the steam with deep breaths for 5 minutes.
2. Use this remedy anytime that you feel nervous.

TIP:

Try lavender essential oil to calm yourself. The smell/odor is very relaxing. You can rub it gently into your temple or put a drop of it on your collarbone to experience a calming effect.

OBSESSIVE COMPULSIVE DISORDER

NATURAL HOME REMEDY

PASSIFLORA & ST JOHN' S WORT

HOW THE REMEDY WORKS

Obsessive compulsive disorder (also known as OCD) is a condition that leads to unwanted repetitive thoughts or actions. OCD affects about 2.2 million American adults. It strikes men and women in roughly equal numbers. If you suffer from OCD, you should seek treatment from your doctor but you can also use this passiflora and St John's wort treatment alongside your doctor's recommendations to reduce the symptoms of OCD in the following ways:

1. **Passiflora:** Passiflora relaxes your mind and can alleviate many of the symptoms of OCD.
2. **St John's Wort**: St John's wort can limit the obsessive thoughts and compulsive behaviors associated with OCD.

HOW TO PREPARE THE REMEDY

1. Add 1 teaspoon of dried passiflora and 1 teaspoon of St John's wort to a cup of hot water and let it steep for 5 minutes.
2. After 5 minutes, strain the water into another cup using a fine mesh strainer and drink it.
3. Drink this remedy up to 4 times per day to manage your OCD.

TIPS:

- People with obsessive compulsive disorder (OCD) often benefit from the nutrients that increase serotonin levels and are likely to reduce symptoms. Try the below tips:
- Stop caffeine drinks completely.
- Ensure you are getting the daily minimum requirement of vitamin B-complex.
- Take 1 tbs. Flax seed oil daily (fatty acids help nourish the nerve sheathing (covering).

OILY SKIN

NATURAL HOME REMEDY

APPLE & CUCUMBER

HOW THE REMEDY WORKS

Oily skin can lead to a range of skin problems including acne and blackheads. Our hormones play a link in the way our oil production glands work. We want to control the oil produced by our skin and at the same time keep our skin hydrated and protected.

This apple and cucumber remedy helps to treat oily skin in the following ways:

1. **Apple:** Apple boosts your skin and helps to regulate the amount oil that gets released onto the skin's surface.
2. **Cucumber:** Cucumber contains a range of nutrients that promote healthy skin and help to remove excess oil.

HOW TO PREPARE THE REMEDY

1. Grate ½ apple and ½ cucumber, mix the shreds together and then use them to cover your oily skin for 10 minutes.
2. After 10 minutes, discard the shreds and wash your skin clean with warm water.
3. Use this remedy daily to treat oily skin.

TIPS:

Lavender is one oily skin treatment that works very well. Lavender has been used for centuries as an antiseptic making it ideal for dealing with pimples and other bacterial infections that are common with oily skin type. Try this:

1. Add 20 drops lavender essential oil to 2 oz of distilled water or witch hazel.
2. Combine ingredients.
3. Store in a glass bottle; with a misting spray top.
4. Spray on skin after washing and let air dry.

Be sure to use sterile containers and keep this mixture in the fridge.

Also See Remedy for Acne and Blackheads in Part 1

ORAL THRUSH

NATURAL HOME REMEDY

APPLE CIDER VINEGAR & TEA TREE OIL

HOW THE REMEDY WORKS

Oral thrush (also known as oral candidiasis) is a fungal yeast infection that affects the lining of the mouth and tongue. When the mouth develops an infection in the mucous membranes, there can be a number of reasons behind it. It can be caused by fungus, by bacteria, or by a disease. One of the more probable causes of mouth infection is the fungus Candida albicans. The yeast infection in the mouth of babies is commonly called thrush while those that occurred in the mouth and throat of adults are referred to as candidiasis or morniliasis Thrush can affect anyone, though it occurs most often in babies and toddlers, older adults, and people with weakened immune systems.

This apple cider vinegar and tea tree oil remedy helps to treat oral thrush in the following ways:

1. **Apple Cider Vinegar:** The enzymes in apple cider vinegar regulate the level of candida (one of the most common causes of oral thrush) in your body.

2. **Tea Tree Oil:** Tea tree oil is a natural disinfectant and helps to treat oral thrush quickly and efficiently.

HOW TO PREPARE THE REMEDY

1. Add 20 drops of tea tree oil and 2 tablespoons of apple cider vinegar to a cup of water and mix well.
2. Gargle this cup of water for 1 minute and then spit it out, *do not swallow.*
3. Use this remedy up to 2 times daily to treat oral thrush.

TIPS:

Prevention:

- The best prevention for thrush is maintaining good oral hygiene by brushing the teeth at least twice a day, flossing at least once a day and using a mouthwash.
- For those using dentures, clean them thoroughly before using.
- For breastfeeding mothers, it's best to have a breast check up for yeast infections.

PIMPLES

NATURAL HOME REMEDY

LEMON JUICE & TEA TREE OIL

HOW THE REMEDY WORKS

Pimples are small, hard spots that appear on the skin as a result of inflammation. Your goal is to keep your pores clear of blockages i.e. preventing the whiteheads and blackheads that lead to pimples. Don't put yourself at risk for developing an infection or scaring. People who are known to touch or pick at their pimples are first advised to stop; this is the best way to keep your skin healthy.

This lemon juice and tea tree oil remedy helps to treat pimples in the following ways:

1. **Lemon Juice:** Lemon juice boosts the skin and clears away pimples.
2. **Tea Tree Oil:** Tea tree oil disinfects and dries out pimples.

HOW TO PREPARE THE REMEDY

1. Soak a cotton ball in lemon juice and then add 5 drops of tea tree oil to the cotton ball.
2. Dab the pimples with the soaked cotton ball.
3. Use this remedy up to 2 times per day until the pimples disappear.

REMEDY VARIATION/TIPS:

Use a Natural Face Mask:

1. **Watercress** contains lots of vitamin A and C and a very healthy addition to your salad or soup. But you can also use it to make a face mask as it is a natural antiseptic.
    - Blend some watercress with plain yogurt and add a couple of spoons of coarse oatmeal.
    - Instead of your usual cleanser, apply some of this mixture with a cotton pad and then gently rinse off residue with warm water.
2. Aloe Vera can also provide relief. When applied to the affected area, Aloe Vera can help to promote healthy healing on the skin.

Also See Remedy for Acne and Blackheads in PART 1

PRE-MENSTRUAL SYNDROME

NATURAL HOME REMEDY

GINKGO BILOBA & LEMON BALM

HOW THE REMEDY WORKS

Premenstrual Syndrome or PMS is a problem that a lot of women wish they could completely block out of their mind. This is because it is a time prior to the menstrual cycle that causes a tremendous amount of frustration and pain each month for a large number of women.
PMS can occur up to 14 days before a woman's menstrual period. It has a wide range of symptoms including anxiety, changes in mood, menstrual cramps and stomach pain.

This ginkgo biloba and lemon balm remedy helps to treat PMS in the following ways:

1. **Ginkgo Biloba:** Ginkgo biloba can reduce the severity of various PMS symptoms.
2. **Lemon Balm:** Lemon balm has a calming effect on the body and can alleviate many PMS symptoms.

HOW TO PREPARE THE REMEDY

1. Add 1 teaspoon of ground ginkgo biloba and 1 teaspoon of ground lemon balm to a cup of boiling water, let it steep for 5 minutes and drink it.
2. Drink this remedy up to 4 times per day when experiencing PMS.

TIPS: More Effective Ways to Treat the Symptoms of PMS Naturally.

Try some of these natural remedies that are known to effectively reduce the symptoms of PMS. Not only are they healthier for the body, they also don't involve any of the harmful side effects that prescription and OTC drugs do.

Below are some healthy natural remedies that have been found to work well at minimizing and sometimes completely eliminating PMS symptoms:

- **Oats** - Not only is this a healthy food product to eat at any time of the day, but it can also help a great deal in lowering the strength of various PMS symptoms.
- **Celery sticks** - Celery sticks are known for being a natural diuretic. This can help to reduce the symptom of boating by enhancing the kidneys function. This in turn causes excess water in the body to be expelled.
- **Apples** - Just about everyone knows that overall health is promoted when a person consumes apples on a regular basis. However, a lot of people are not aware that they can also reduce swelling that commonly occurs with PMS.

- **Massage** - The abdominal pain associated with premenstrual syndrome can be reduced by simply enjoying a massage with the use of **essential oils like sage and lavender.**
- **Barley water** - Drinking barley water is a natural and healthy way to reduce the discomfort that goes along with many of the PMS symptoms.
- **Calcium** - It is common for calcium levels in a woman's body to be lower during menstruation. For this reason, it is important to increase the level of calcium in the diet, and it can also be beneficial to take calcium supplements.
- **Evening primrose oil** - Numerous women have been taking evening primrose oil for many years to reduce the pain and discomfort caused from PMS. It is a natural herbal remedy that is well-known to be effective for the treatment of PMS.

PSORIASIS

NATURAL HOME REMEDY

APPLE CIDER VINEGAR & COLLOIDAL OATMEAL

HOW THE REMEDY WORKS

Psoriasis is a skin disorder that leads to flaky skin, itching, redness and pain. Psoriasis causes cells to build up rapidly on the surface of the skin. The extra skin cells form thick, silvery scales and itchy, dry, red patches that are sometimes painful. There are quite a few natural remedies that are used today to relieve the bothersome symptoms of psoriasis. Below are a few natural treatment options that have proven to be effective at relieving the itchy flakiness of this skin condition.

This apple cider vinegar and colloidal oatmeal remedy helps to treat psoriasis in the following ways:

1. **Apple Cider Vinegar:** Inflammation of the skin has been treated for many years with the use of apple cider vinegar. Apple cider vinegar neutralizes your skin and protects against the itching and irritation caused by psoriasis. One of the reasons it is believed to be so effective at relieving the

itching of psoriasis is because of its antibacterial properties. Its benefits have even been recognized by the Psoriasis Foundation for the help it provides to those suffering with the symptoms of psoriasis.

2. **Colloidal Oatmeal:** Colloidal oatmeal hydrates and moisturizes the skin which helps to combat psoriasis.

HOW TO PREPARE THE REMEDY

1. Add 1 cup of apple cider vinegar and 1 cup of colloidal oatmeal to a hot bath and soak in it for up to 30 minutes.
2. Use this remedy up to 3 times per week to treat psoriasis.

REMEDY VARIATIONS

1. **Apple cider vinegar** - To make a natural treatment that is soothing to the skin add one cup of apple cider vinegar to a gallon of water. Soak a washcloth with this solution then gently rub on the affected area to decrease itching.
2. **Heated olive oil** – Scalp flakiness is a frequent problem psoriasis sufferers find themselves dealing with on a regular basis. This is an issue that can naturally cause many uncomfortable and embarrassing moments. Warm olive oil is a natural home remedy that can help to resolve issues with itching, psoriasis scales, and scalp flakiness. Simply heat a small amount of olive oil in a pan, being careful not to get it too hot. Next, dip the fingertips into the olive oil and gently massage into all areas of the scalp. Let it remain on the scalp for a couple minutes, then wash away using a mild shampoo.

3. **Baking soda** - Baking soda is another home remedy that has been used for years to relieve the symptoms of many skin conditions. It works great for relieving the symptom of itching that psoriasis is known for causing. Mix half a glass baking soda with one gallon water and massage into the scalp or apply to other affected areas of the skin using a clean washcloth.
4. **Epsom salts** - The use of Epsom salts is a natural remedy that is well known for being able to provide relief for a wide variety of different ailments. When added to bath water, the healing powers of these therapeutic salts quickly go to work. Not only are they helpful for decreasing itching, but they also work at reducing swelling as well.
5. **Dead Sea salt** - This is another natural remedy that helps to prolong the remission of psoriasis outbreaks and reduces swelling when added to bath water.

PART 4: Q THRU Z

"Wherever the art of medicine is loved, there is also a love of humanity."

Hippocrates

QUEASINESS

NATURAL HOME REMEDY

FENNEL SEEDS & GINGER

HOW THE REMEDY WORKS

Queasiness is a feeling of mild sickness that is similar to nausea. The sick to the stomach feeling that precedes vomiting.

This fennel seeds and ginger remedy helps to treat queasiness in the following ways:

1. **Fennel Seeds:** Fennel seeds calm your stomach and combat the inflammation that can cause queasiness.
2. **Ginger:** Ginger has a positive effect on your intestines and stomach and helps to relieve any feelings of queasiness.

HOW TO PREPARE THE REMEDY

1. Add 1 teaspoon of ground fennel seeds and 1 teaspoon of ground ginger to a cup of hot water, let it steep for 5 minutes and drink it.

2. Drink this remedy up to 4 times per day to treat queasiness.

TIPS:

1. When you start feeling queasiness, lie or sit down; this will help settle your stomach.
2. Baking Soda &Water: This solution gives relief from bloating, stomach acid and queasiness.
   - Take 1/2 glass of water and dissolve 1 teaspoon of baking soda in it.
   - Stir it well till the baking soda is dissolved, drink. It will help settle the queasiness and gas.
3. Do not eat spicy foods till the queasiness problem passes, eat light foods such as oatmeal or crackers instead.

Also see Remedy for Nausea in Part 3

RASHES

NATURAL HOME REMEDY

BAKING SODA & COCONUT OIL

HOW THE REMEDY WORKS

Rashes are red, inflamed, itchy sections that develop on the skin for various reasons. A rash can refer to many different skin conditions; and can be caused, directly or indirectly, by a bacterial, viral, or fungal infection.

This baking soda and coconut oil remedy helps to treat rashes in the following ways:

1. **Baking Soda:** Baking soda repairs the damage caused by rashes.
2. **Coconut Oil:** Coconut oil is a potent moisturizer that soothes rashes on the skin.

HOW TO PREPARE THE REMEDY

1. Mix 1 teaspoon of baking soda with 2 tablespoons of coconut oil to form a paste.
2. Apply this paste to the rash for 5 minutes and then wash it clean with warm water.
3. Use this remedy daily until the rash disappears.

REMEDY VARIATIONS/TIP:

1. **Coconut oil** can be added to cumin seeds to prepare a paste. This mixture should be applied in thick layers to the affected area approximately one hour before a bath or shower.
2. **Soak** in a tub of lukewarm water that you have added ground oatmeal powder and baking soda.

Effective Treatment Options for Heat Rash:
Heat rash is a skin problem that can be extremely uncomfortable and it can also cause sensations where the skin either itches or burns. During the summer months when the days are hot there are frequently a large number of infants, children, and adults that deal with the bothersome symptoms of heat rash.

Here's good news! There are several different natural treatments for heat rash that work very well. A few of these are as follows:

- **Avocado** – This is a fruit that is a great tasting source of both linoleic acid and vitamin E. One of the great things about avocados is the natural healing properties that they contain, and they also help a great deal in soothing the irritation of heat rash. The linoleic acid in avocados promotes the regeneration process of the skin. Vitamin E helps to form a coating on the cells of the skin and it also aids in the process of dead skin cells falling off.

- **Aloe Vera** - This is an herbal remedy that can help in the treatment of a wide range of different conditions of the skin. It helps to promote healing and it works great in soothing irritated skin. Aloe Vera is also used to reduce the symptom of itching that heat rash commonly causes. The antibiotic properties that this herb contains are what cause it to be such a good treatment option for heat rash and various other skin conditions.
- **Lavender** - Heat rash is a condition of the skin that is known to cause inflammation. Lavender contains antibacterial and soothing properties that quickly go to work reducing inflammation of the skin. Due to its antibacterial properties it is also a great natural herbal remedy that can be used for the prevention of heat rash.
- **Oil of Peppermint** - This is a natural herbal remedy that works rather quickly in soothing the irritation of heat rash. As an added benefit, oil of peppermint also contains antibiotic and antibacterial properties as well. This means that not only is it a great treatment option for soothing and reducing the discomfort caused by heat rash, but it also works to heal this type of skin rash as well.

RESTLESS LEG SYNDROME

NATURAL HOME REMEDY

ALMOND OIL & LAVENDER OIL

HOW THE REMEDY WORKS

Restless leg syndrome (also known as RLS) is a disorder characterized by throbbing, pulling, creeping, or other unpleasant sensations in the legs and an uncontrollable, and sometimes overwhelming, urge to move them. RLS is a common problem with one in ten people suffering from its symptoms. RLS occurs in both men and women, although the occurrence is about twice as high in women. Symptoms occur primarily at night when a person is relaxing or at rest and can increase in severity during the night. Moving the legs relieves the discomfort.

This almond oil and lavender oil remedy may also help to relieve RLS in the following ways:

1. **Almond Oil:** Almond oil is a natural relaxant and can reduce the sensations associated with Restless Leg Syndrome.

2. **Lavender Oil:** Lavender oil naturally relieves the itchiness and tingling that often comes with Restless Leg Syndrome.

HOW TO PREPARE THE REMEDY

1. Mix 5 drops of lavender oil with 2 tablespoons of almond oil.
2. Massage this mixture into your legs for 5 minutes and then wash them clean with warm water.
3. Use this remedy daily to treat Restless Leg Syndrome.

TIPS:

RLS is different from other ailments as the exact nature of its origin is still not fully understood. It was earlier thought that RLS is purely a neurological problem and medication is the only treatment. However, various studies in this field have shown that there are a number of contributing factors leading to this condition.

One of the main factors responsible for RLS is the deficiency of certain vital minerals such as iron, folate and magnesium in the body. It is therefore important to eat a wide ranging diet in all essential nutrients; include a lot of leafy vegetables such as spinach and fruits like apples. Alcohol, caffeine and other stimulants are also known to aggravate the symptoms.

The most common feature in this condition is an irresistible urge to move the body as it provides immediate relief from the unpleasant sensations. It has been found that some form of regular exercise is beneficial.

There are many light exercises you can try to get immediate as well as long term relief from RLS symptoms.

Any exercise routine should include walking as it tones up the muscles of entire body and promotes blood circulation. In addition, one may incorporate stretching as well as aerobic exercises. Before going to bed, some calf stretches are helpful to relieve stress from legs and reduce night time jerking and disruption of sleep.

RINGWORM

NATURAL HOME REMEDY

NEEM OIL & TEA TREE OIL

HOW THE REMEDY WORKS

Ringworm is a fungal infection that causes ring shaped scaly patches to form on the skin. Some people believe the ringworm rash is actually caused from a worm; this is far from being the truth. It is a fungal infection that can occur on various parts of the body and it is caused by dermatophytes that live on the outer layer of human skin.

The ringworm infection is known to thrive in moist warm areas on the body. The treatment of the ringworm rash is frequently quite easy and it usually does not require a visit to a health care professional. There are natural alternative treatments that can be found at home.

This neem oil and tea tree oil remedy helps to treat ringworm in the following ways:

1. **Neem Oil:** Neem oil is a powerful antifungal which destroys the fungi that cause ringworm.

2. **Tea Tree Oil:** Tea tree oil is a natural remedy that has become known for being very effective at killing the germ causing this type of fungal infection. Tea tree oil disinfects the skin affected by ringworm.

HOW TO PREPARE THE REMEDY

1. Add 5 drops of neem oil and 5 drops of tea tree oil to a cotton ball.
2. Wipe the affected skin with the cotton ball.
3. Use this remedy up to 2 times per day until the ringworm disappears.

REMEDY VARIATIONS:

Some of the other natural remedies found in most any home include:

1. **Garlic, Lemon, Iodine, Olive oil, and Vinegar.** Each of these is very inexpensive treatment options. When one of these home remedies is used, gently rub it onto the affected area of the skin (use cotton ball).
2. **Papaya** is another natural remedy that can relieve the symptoms caused by the ringworm infection.

These treatment options have proven to work very well at clearing up the ringworm infection and decreasing the common symptom of itching it often causes.

RUNNY NOSE

NATURAL HOME REMEDY

EUCALYPTUS OIL & ROSEMARY OIL

HOW THE REMEDY WORKS

A runny nose occurs when the nasal passages and sinuses get filled with excess mucus. The drainage of a runny nose may run out of your nose or down the back of your throat or both. A runny nose is especially common during winter, and also could be caused by an infection (like a cold or the flu) or by allergies, crying, irritating smells, or particles in the air.

This eucalyptus oil and rosemary oil remedy helps to treat a runny nose in the following ways:

1. **Eucalyptus Oil:** Eucalyptus oil flushes mucus out of the sinuses and nasal passages.
2. **Rosemary Oil:** Rosemary oil eases the inflammation that causes a runny nose.

HOW TO PREPARE THE REMEDY

1. Put 5 drops of eucalyptus oil and 5 drops of rosemary oil on a paper towel and then place it on your pillow while you sleep.
2. When you wake up, discard the paper towel, add 5 drops of eucalyptus oil and 5 drops of rosemary oil to a bowl of boiling water and breathe in the steam with deep breaths for 5 minutes.
3. Use this remedy daily until the runny nose subsides.

REMEDY VARIATIONS:

Ginger has various antioxidants along with antiviral and anti-bacterial properties. It will help loosen phlegm and also give relief from respiratory discomforts. Ginger is good for runny nose and others symptoms of cold and flu i.e. sore throat and fever etc**. Drink Ginger Tea for Runny Nose:**

- Take 1-2 inch piece of fresh ginger and cut it into slices. Place these slices in a cup and pour hot water over it.
- Let steep for about 10 minutes. Strain and add 1 tsp honey (optional) and drink it.

Drink Sage Tea for Runny Nose:

This is one of the most effective herbal remedies for runny nose and related infections. Sage has anti-bacterial and anti-inflammatory properties.

- Use 1 tsp dried sage leaves, 1 cup of hot water, 1 tsp honey (optional) Place sage in a pot, pour hot water over it.
- Let steep for 5-8 minutes. Strain and add honey if using.
- Drink this tea once a day to relieve runny nose.

SHINGLES

NATURAL HOME REMEDY

GARLIC & LICORICE

HOW THE REMEDY WORKS

Shingles is an inflammatory viral infection that causes a red blistering rash to form on the skin. Shingles is caused by the same virus that causes chickenpox. Shingles can occur anywhere on your body, it most often appears as a single stripe of blisters that wraps around either the left or the right side of your torso. Shingles most commonly affects older adults and people with weak immune systems.

This garlic and licorice remedy helps to treat shingles in the following ways:

1. **Garlic:** Garlic's anti-inflammatory and antiviral properties help to treat shingles and reduce the painful associated symptoms.
2. **Licorice:** Licorice is also a potent antiviral that directly combats shingles.

HOW TO PREPARE THE REMEDY

1. Crush 2 garlic cloves using a mortar and pestle.
2. Mix these ground garlic cloves with 1 teaspoon of licorice powder and a small amount of water to form a paste.
3. Apply the paste to the shingles for 5 minutes and then wash it clean with warm water.
4. Use this remedy up to 2 times per day until the shingles subsides.

REMEDY VARIATION/TIPS:

Aloe Vera and Shingles: Aloe Vera has been used to treat skin problems for many years...

Aloe Vera is known to be one of the excellent herbal cures for shingles. The anti inflammatory properties of this herb are proved to be practical in reducing the pain as well as clearing the blisters caused due to shingles
Aloe is a succulent plant with a cool, gooey interior. The best way to use aloe to treat your shingles is to obtain a real aloe plant.

- Cut the leaves off the plant, cut each leaf in half lengthwise to maximize the surface area of the gel.
- Scrape the gel out of the leaf and apply aloe gel over the blisters and affected area of the skin.
- Apply the gel to the skin as often as you want.

Remember: It is important to maintain good personal hygiene, avoid scratching, and try to keep the affected area clean in order to prevent a secondary bacterial infection of the skin.

SINUS INFECTION

NATURAL HOME REMEDY

GARLIC & OREGANO OIL

HOW THE REMEDY WORKS

Sinus infections (sinusitis) cause swelling, inflammation and blockages in your sinuses. Sinusitis is inflammation of the air cavities within the passages of the nose. Sinusitis can be caused by infection, but also can be caused by allergies and chemical or particulate irritation of the sinuses. Sinus infection symptoms may include sinus headache, facial tenderness, pressure or pain in the sinuses, fever, cloudy discolored drainage, and feeling of nasal stuffiness, sore throat, and cough, and on rare occasions, associated with facial swelling.

This garlic and oregano oil remedy helps to treat sinus infections in the following ways:

1. **Garlic:** Garlic fights the inflammation associated with sinus infections and helps to reduce any blockages and swelling.

2. **Oregano Oil:** Oregano oil clears your sinuses and also boosts your immune system which helps to speed up your sinus infection recovery.

HOW TO PREPARE THE REMEDY

1. Put 5 drops of oregano oil on a paper towel and then place it on your pillow while you sleep.

2. When you wake up, discard the paper towel, add 3 cloves of garlic and 5 drops of oregano oil to a bowl of boiling water and breathe in the steam with deep breaths for 5 minutes.

3. Use this remedy daily until the sinus infection subsides.

REMEDY VARIATION:

Peppermint is another herb that is often used as tea to calm irritated nasal membrane. The leaves are steep in hot water for 10 minutes to release the menthol oil which has a strong decongestant effect.

1. Use 1 peppermint teabags or 1 heaping teaspoons of dried peppermint loose-leaf tea, or a handful (1 - 2 stalks) of fresh, blemish-free peppermint leaves.
2. 8 oz. fresh, water, brought just to the boil. Add (optional) honey, and lemon or lime.
3. Cool the just-boiled water slightly (herbal teas are best when steeped in hot, steamy - but not boiling - water), and then add to your cup.
4. Cover peppermint tea and let it steep for10 minutes (herbal teas improve with longer steeping times - their flavor is enhanced and you'll enjoy their fullest health benefits!).
5. Remove the teabag or tea leaves from your cup and enjoy.

Remember to brew fresh leaves a minute or two longer than dried leaves or a teabag.

SLEEP PROBLEMS

NATURAL HOME REMEDY

CHAMOMILE & VALERIAN

HOW THE REMEDY WORKS

Sleep problems can be caused by illness, medications or stress. Sleep is so important and not sleeping enough can affect your life in so many ways. This includes not being able to lose weight and not having enough energy to get through each day. Lack of sleep often results in mood swings. You may find that you become irritable, impatience, moody and that your concentration levels disappear. This chamomile and valerian remedy helps to treat sleep problems in the following ways:

1. **Chamomile:** Chamomile is a natural relaxant and makes it easy to fall into a deep, restful sleep.
2. **Valerian:** Valerian is a natural sedative and helps to relax your body and mind before you sleep.

HOW TO PREPARE THE REMEDY

1. Add 1 teaspoon of dried chamomile and 1 teaspoon of dried valerian root to a cup of hot water and let it steep for 5 minutes.

2. After 5 minutes, strain the water into another cup using a fine mesh strainer and drink it.
3. Drink this remedy each night 1 hour before you sleep to enhance your sleep quality.

Also See Insomnia in Part 2

REMEDY VARIATION/TIPS:

Lemon Balm - In contrast to valerian, lemon balm tastes very good and makes a lemony tea. Like chamomile, drinking a cup in the evenings may help promote sleep. You could mix it with chamomile tea as well.

FOODS:

Magnesium-containing foods, such as almonds, seeds, black beans, salmon, dark leafy greens and most whole grains are helpful (although if beans give you uncomfortable gas, they should probably be avoided). Magnesium is crucial to muscle and nerve function, particularly muscle relaxation.

Whole grains and other complex carbohydrates may also promote sleep, as they are said to stimulate serotonin in the brain.

Plain, low-fat yogurt with raw honey makes a good bedtime snack. Raw honey is actually alleged to promote sleep and even weight loss, while yogurt contains calcium, which is also important to muscle relaxation. Calcium also helps with melatonin production in the body.

SNORING

NATURAL HOME REMEDY

PEPPERMINT OIL & TEA TREE OIL

HOW THE REMEDY WORKS

Snoring is an irritating disorder that can disrupt your sleep patterns and the sleep patterns of those around you. It is a common problem among all ages and both genders. According to the National Sleep Foundation; snoring affects approximately 90 million American adults – 37 million on a regular basis. Snoring may occur nightly or intermittently. Persons most at risk are males and those who are overweight. Snoring occurs when air flows past relaxed tissues in your throat, causing the tissues to vibrate as you breathe, which creates those irritating sounds.

This peppermint oil and tea tree oil remedy helps to treat snoring in the following ways:

1. **Peppermint Oil:** Peppermint oil soothes the inflammation in the nostrils and throat which often leads to snoring.
2. **Tea Tree Oil:** Tea tree oil opens up your throat and nostrils and promotes proper breathing which helps to eliminate snoring.

HOW TO PREPARE THE REMEDY

1. Put 5 drops of peppermint oil and 5 drops of tea tree oil on a paper towel and then place it on your pillow while you sleep.
2. When you wake up, discard the paper towel, add 5 drops of peppermint oil and 5 drops of tea tree oil to a bowl of boiling water and breathe in the steam with deep breaths for 5 minutes.
3. Use this remedy daily to treat snoring.

TIPS:

People who snore make a vibrating, rattling, noisy sound while breathing during sleep. It may be a symptom of sleep apnea. Consult your doctor if you snore and have any of the following symptoms or signs:

- Excessive daytime sleepiness
- Morning headaches
- Recent weight gain
- Awakening in the morning not feeling rested
- Awaking at night feeling confused
- Change in your level of attention, concentration, or memory
- Observed pauses in breathing during sleep

SORE THROATS

NATURAL HOME REMEDY

LICORICE

HOW THE REMEDY WORKS

Licorice was a popular natural remedy among the ancient Chinese and Egyptians who both used it to cure a wide range of ailments. It was first referenced as a natural remedy for sore throats by the Greek philosopher Theophrastus, who stated it was good for coughs in his book 'Enquiry into Plants' which was written between 350 BC & 287 BC.

Licorice is a potent anti-inflammatory and antiviral. This allows it to prevent the growth of viral infections that often cause sore throats and also reduce any pain or swelling around the throat. While licorice is a fantastic choice for soothing sore throats, many products marketed as licorice in the US are actually made from anise oil and contain little or no licorice. Therefore, you need to make sure you check the ingredients of any licorice product you buy and confirm that it contains genuine licorice before preparing this natural sore throat remedy.

HOW TO PREPARE THE REMEDY

There are lots of ways to use licorice as a treatment for sore throats and one of the best is licorice root tea. To prepare licorice root tea, follow the instructions below:

1. Boil 8 oz. of water in a saucepan.
2. When the water starts to boil, remove the saucepan from the heat and add 2 teaspoons of licorice root to the water. Let the licorice root steep in the water for 5 minutes, then strain the licorice root tea into a cup using a fine mesh strainer and drink it.

TIPS: SIDE EFFECTS

For the best results with this licorice root tea sore throat remedy, drink it up to 3 times per day. It's important that you drink no more than 3 cups of licorice root tea each day or you may experience unpleasant side effects such as fatigue, headaches, muscle pain and numbness.
Note: Check with your doctor before using licorice if you are taking any medications.

REMEDY VARIATIONS:

To increase the potency of this licorice root tea and get rid of your sore throat even faster, try mixing it with the following natural sore throat remedies:

1. **Cinnamon**: Cinnamon combats the bacteria that lead to sore throats and also enhances the flow of blood to your throat

which helps to fight the infection. To soothe your sore throat with cinnamon and licorice root tea, add a teaspoon of cinnamon powder to the licorice root tea, mix it well and drink it.

2. **Lemon:** Lemon is a powerful immune system booster that helps your body fight infections such as sore throats and also helps to remove mucus from the throat. To soothe your sore throat with lemon and licorice tea, squeeze the juice from half a lemon into the licorice tea, mix it well and drink it.
3. **Marshmallow Root:** Marshmallow root contains mucilage - a substance that forms into a gel like substance which then coats and soothes your sore throat. To soothe your sore throat with marshmallow root and licorice root, boil 8 oz. of water in a saucepan and then when the water starts to boil, remove the saucepan from the heat and add 2 teaspoons of licorice root and 2 teaspoons of marshmallow root to the water. Let the mixture steep for 10 minutes, then strain the marshmallow and licorice root tea into a cup using a fine mesh strainer and drink it.
4. **Turmeric:** Turmeric has anti-inflammatory and antiseptic properties which help to heal your sore throat faster and also reduce any discomfort you may experience. To soothe your sore throat with turmeric and licorice tea, add half a teaspoon of turmeric powder to the licorice root tea, mix it well and drink it.

STOMACH ULCERS

NATURAL HOME REMEDY

BANANA & COCONUT MILK

HOW THE REMEDY WORKS

Stomach ulcers (also known as peptic ulcers) are painful open sores or raw area in the lining of the stomach. The word "peptic" means that the cause of the problem is due to acid. The two most common types of peptic ulcer are called "gastric ulcers" and "duodenal ulcers". These names refer to the location where the ulcer is found. Gastric ulcers are located in the stomach. Duodenal ulcers are found at the beginning of the small intestine (also called the small bowel). A person may have both gastric and duodenal ulcers at the same time. A burning stomach pain is the most common symptom.

This banana and coconut milk remedy helps to treat stomach ulcers in the following ways:

1. **Banana:** Banana prevents the growth of various bacteria that cause stomach ulcers. Bananas will neutralize the over-acidity of the gastric juices and it will also lessen the ulcer's irritation by coating the stomach lining.

2. **Coconut Milk**: Coconut milk has a soothing effect on stomach ulcers and relieves their painful symptoms.

HOW TO PREPARE THE REMEDY

1. Blend 1 banana and 1 cup of coconut milk in a blender until smooth and then drink it.
2. Drink this remedy up to 2 times per day until the stomach ulcer subsides.

TIPS:

Avoid foods and drinks that cause discomfort for you. For many people these include alcohol, coffee, caffeinated soda, fatty foods, chocolate, and spicy foods.

- Avoid eating late night snacks.
- Reduce your stress level and learn ways to better manage stress.
- Quit smoking (and all tobacco products).
- Avoid drugs such as aspirin, ibuprofen (Advil, Motrin), or naproxen (Aleve, Naprosyn).
- Check with your healthcare provider, stomach ulcers are often a side effect of pain killers and anti-inflammatory drugs.

TENDONITIS

NATURAL HOME REMEDY

CAYENNE & EXTRA VIRGIN OLIVE OIL

HOW THE REMEDY WORKS

Tendonitis is a condition that develops when your tendons become inflamed. It can cause pain, redness and swelling in the affected area. Tendonitis is mostly caused by overusing a tendon or injuring it; and can affect people of any age, but is more common among adults who participate in a lot of sports. Tendonitis can occur in various parts of the body, including the elbow, wrist, finger, or thigh. Elderly individuals are also susceptible to tendonitis because our tendons tend to lose their elasticity and become weaker as we get older.

Here are some activities that can cause tendonitis:

- Gardening - Shoveling - Painting - Tennis - Golf -
- Throwing and pitching ball.
- Also incorrect posture at work or home or poor stretching before exercise or playing sports increases a person's risk of tendonitis.

This cayenne and extra virgin olive oil remedy helps to treat tendonitis in the following ways:

1. **Cayenne:** Cayenne's pain relieving and warming properties help to soothe tendonitis.
2. **Extra Virgin Olive Oil:** Extra virgin olive oil stimulates blood flow, reduces pain and speeds up your recovery from tendonitis.

HOW TO PREPARE THE REMEDY

1. Warm ½ cup of extra virgin olive oil in a saucepan, then add 1 tablespoon of cayenne powder and mix it well.
2. Massage the mixture into the affected tendons, leave it on for 30 minutes and then wash it clean with warm water.
3. Use this remedy up to 4 times per day to treat tendonitis.

TIPS:

Things you can do to help prevent tendonitis:

- Stop doing the activity that caused the tendonitis; you need to rest the injury.
- Before exercising, warm up thoroughly, gradually building the intensity level of your workout. Cool down after the session.
- Train for a new sport before you start it. Start building strength and flexibility in the muscles you will use a few weeks or months in advance.

TOOTHACHE

NATURAL HOME REMEDY

BLACK PEPPER GARLIC & SEA SALT

HOW THE REMEDY WORKS

Toothache can be caused by various things and can range from a slight soreness in the teeth or gums to an intense pain in these areas.
This black pepper, garlic and sea salt remedy helps to treat toothache in the following ways:

1. **Black Pepper:** Black pepper has natural pain relieving properties and can instantly reduce toothache.
2. **Garlic:** Garlic directly targets the pain associated with toothache and helps you to recover from it at a faster rate.
3. **Sea Salt:** Sea salt combats many of the infections that cause toothache.

HOW TO PREPARE THE REMEDY

1. Mix 1 crushed garlic clove with 1 teaspoon of black pepper and 1 teaspoon of sea salt, then apply it directly to the affected tooth or teeth for 5 minutes.
2. After 5 minutes, rinse your mouth out with water or mouthwash and brush your teeth.
3. Use this remedy up to 4 times per day until the toothache subsides.

REMEDY VARIATION/TIP:

Use Clove Oil

Clove works at relieving tooth pain and decreasing infection. Cloves contain a natural anesthetic called eugenol, which numbs whatever it comes in contact with:

- Either chew one or apply clove oil to the hurting area.

- Put one or two drops of the oil onto cotton ball and apply it to the throbbing tooth.

Clove oil may numb the affected area temporarily; it is short-term relief until you can see your dentist.

UPSET STOMACH

NATURAL HOME REMEDY

APPLE CIDER VINEGAR & GINGER

HOW THE REMEDY WORKS

An upset stomach is an unpleasant condition that can cause bloating, diarrhea and stomach pain. There are many causes for an upset stomach, including food poisoning, an infection, overeating, too much stress, excessive drinking, motion sickness, a side effect of medication, a gastrointestinal disease.

This apple cider vinegar and ginger remedy helps to treat an upset stomach in the following ways:

1. **Apple Cider** Vinegar: Apple cider vinegar boosts your digestive system and calms your stomach.
2. **Ginger:** ginger provides relief for a variety of stomach ailments. In particular, ginger is helpful in relieving nausea and vomiting. Ginger combats many of the bacteria that cause an upset stomach.

HOW TO PREPARE THE REMEDY

1. Add 1 tablespoon of apple cider vinegar and 1 teaspoon of ground ginger to a cup of hot water, mix well and drink it.
2. Drink this remedy up to 4 times per day until the upset stomach subsides.

REMEDY VARIATION:

Peppermint calms the muscles of the stomach and improves the flow of bile, which the body uses to digest fats. Peppermint also relaxes the muscles that allow painful digestive gas to pass. Herbal teas, such as peppermint tea, can soothe your upset stomach.

Peppermint Tea:

- Use a tea bag or steep 1 tsp. dried peppermint leaves in 1 cup boiling water for 10 minutes; strain and cool.
- Drink 4 to 5 times per day between meals until the upset stomach is gone.

URINARY TRACT INFECTION

NATURAL HOME REMEDY

BAKING SODA

HOW THE REMEDY WORKS

Urinary Tract Infections (also known as UTIs) are a type of bladder infection that affect both men and women but are 10 times more common among females, with the lifetime risk for a woman of contracting a UTI estimated to be between 40% and 50%. The symptoms of urinary tract infection may include:

- Back pain
- Blood in the urine
- Cloudy urine
- Increased frequency of urination
- Light pain or discomfort in the pubic region
- Pain or a burning feeling during urination

Baking soda helps to treat UTIs naturally by neutralizing the acidity of your urine.
This relieves many of the painful symptoms of UTIs listed above and also allows your body to fight the infection and recover more quickly.

HOW TO PREPARE THE REMEDY

1. Baking soda is most commonly consumed in liquid form. To prepare a liquid based natural UTI remedy with baking soda, follow the instructions below:
2. Add ½ teaspoon of baking soda to 1 cup of cold water.
3. Mix the baking soda and cold water together thoroughly and then drink immediately.

TIPS:

Caution: For the best results with this natural UTI remedy, drink it twice daily for up to 2 days. If after 2 days the UTI has not subsided, you will need to seek medical attention to ensure that it does not enter your bloodstream or spread to your kidneys. Also, make sure you consume this natural UTI remedy at least 1 hour after eating. Ingesting baking soda when your stomach is full can lead to severe stomach pain.

REMEDY VARIATIONS:

To maximize your UTI recovery, you can also try the following natural UTI remedy variations which combine baking soda with other natural UTI fighting ingredients:

1. **Apple Cider Vinegar:** Apple cider vinegar is packed full of enzymes and minerals that naturally fight bacteria and can help you recover from UTIs faster. To treat your UTI with apple cider vinegar and baking soda, combine 2 tablespoons of apple cider vinegar and ½ teaspoon of baking soda with a

cup of boiling water and drink it twice daily for up to 2 days.

2. **Blueberry Juice:** Blueberry juice is packed full of antibacterial phytonutrients that can help to contain and treat your UTI. To treat your UTI with blueberries and baking soda, combine ½ teaspoon of baking soda with a glass of blueberry juice and drink it twice daily for up to 2 days.
3. **Cranberry Juice:** Cranberry juice contains various compounds that protect your urinary tract against bacteria and reduce your risk of contracting a UTI. To treat your UTI with cranberry juice and baking soda, combine ½ teaspoon of baking soda with a glass of cranberry juice and drink it twice daily for up to 2 days.
4. **Pineapple Juice:** Fresh pineapple juice contains an enzyme called bromelain which has anti-inflammatory properties and can help soothe the painful symptoms associated with UTIs. To treat your UTI with pineapple juice and baking soda, combine ½ teaspoon of baking soda with a glass of pineapple juice and drink it twice daily for up to 2 days.

VAGINAL INFECTION

NATURAL HOME REMEDY

TEA TREE OIL & YOGURT

HOW THE REMEDY WORKS

Vaginal Infection (also known as vaginitis) Vaginitis is a medical term used to describe various conditions that cause infection or inflammation of the vagina.

Vaginal infections have a range of possible symptoms including:

- A burning sensation while urinating, vaginal discharge and itching around the vagina.
- Abnormal vaginal discharge with an unpleasant odor.
- Discomfort during intercourse.

The six most common types of vaginal infections are:

1. Candida or Yeast Infections (See Remedy for Yeast Infection)
2. Bacterial vaginosis.
3. Trichomoniasis vaginitis.
4. Chlamydia vaginitis.
5. Viral vaginitis.
6. Non-infectious vaginitis.

This manuka honey and yogurt remedy helps to treat vaginal infections in the following ways:

1. **Tea Tree Oil:** Tea tree oil fights many vaginal infections and speeds up your recovery.
2. **Yogurt:** Probiotic yogurts prevent the growth of the fungus that causes vaginal yeast infections.

HOW TO PREPARE THE REMEDY

1. Add 2 drops of tea tree oil to a fresh tampon then dip the tampon in probiotic yogurt and insert it into your vagina.
2. Replace the tampon and repeat this remedy 2 times per day until the vaginal infection subsides.

TIPS:

- To prevent vaginal yeast infection from occurring, avoid using douches, feminine sprays, scented toilet paper and deodorant tampons.
- It is also best to wear cotton underwear and avoid wearing tight pants or panty hoses.
- When wearing a wet suit or a bathing suit, it is recommended to change out of it right away.

VERTIGO

NATURAL HOME REMEDY

BASIL & CORIANDER SEEDS

HOW THE REMEDY WORKS

Vertigo is a sensation that can cause dizziness, loss of balance, nausea and ringing in the ears. A sensation of dizziness marked by the feeling that one's self or surroundings are spinning or whirling. What Causes a Person to Suffer From Vertigo?
The two main kinds of vertigo are central and peripheral. Peripheral vertigo occurs from a problem with a person's vestibular system. The vestibular system includes the vestibular nerve and inner ear and it controls balance. Central vertigo is the result of problems related to a person's brain. In some cases a person may never know the cause of why they suffer from vertigo
This basil and coriander seeds remedy helps to treat vertigo in the following ways:

1. **Basil:** Basil helps you feel more coordinated and alleviates many of the symptoms of vertigo.
2. **Coriander Seeds:** Coriander seeds are one of the most popular natural ingredients for fighting vertigo.

HOW TO PREPARE THE REMEDY

1. Add 1 teaspoon of ground basil and 1 teaspoon of ground coriander seeds to a cup of hot water, let it steep for 5 minutes and drink it.
2. Drink this remedy up to 4 times per day to treat vertigo...

TIPS:

Often vertigo can accompany other symptoms which can vary depending on the condition or disease. Symptoms that frequently affect a person's vestibular system might also involve other body systems - these include:

- Lightheadedness
- Blurred/double vision
- Dizziness
- Impaired coordination/balance
- Nausea with or without vomiting
- Tinnitus

Some less common symptoms that can occur with vertigo may include:

- Slurred speech
- Difficulty swallowing
- Abnormal movements of the eyes
- Loss of consciousness/confusions for even a brief moment
- Progressive numbness/weakness in the arms/legs
- Changes in taste, smell, or hearing
- Facial paralysis/weakness
- Difficulty focusing the eyes

NOTE: There are many causes of both types of vertigo and in some cases there are no known causes. It may be temporary or long-term depending on the underlying cause.

If you are experiencing other serious symptoms, such as abnormal behavior, severe headache, changes in consciousness, and vomiting you should seek immediate medical care.

VITILIGO

NATURAL ~ HOME REMEDY

BAKUCHI OIL & COCONUT OIL

HOW THE REMEDY WORKS

Vitiligo is a common, autoimmune skin disease in which there is loss of pigment from areas of the skin resulting in irregular white spots or patches. These patches are more common in areas where the skin is exposed to the sun. The skin has normal texture. Vitiligo may appear at any age. The patches may be on the hands, feet, arms, face, and lips. Other common areas for white patches are:

- The armpits and groin (where the leg meets the body)
- Around the mouth
- Eyes, Nostrils, Navel,
- Genitals and Rectal areas.

According to The National Institute of Arthritis and Musculoskeletal and Skin Diseases (NIH) one to two million people in the United States have this skin disorder! The disorder affects all races, both male and female equally. Vitiligo is not contagious in any way.

This bakuchi oil and coconut oil remedy helps to treat vitiligo in the following ways:

1. **Bakuchi Oil:** Bakuchi oil contains various components that restore color to white patches on the skin. Also used to treat a variety of skin problems.
2. **Coconut Oil:** Coconut oil stimulates repigmentation of the skin.

HOW TO PREPARE THE REMEDY

1. Mix 2 tablespoons of bakuchi oil and 2 tablespoons of coconut oil in a bowl and then massage this mixture directly into the white patches of skin.
2. Use this remedy up to 4 times per day until the white patches disappear.

TIPS:

Protect your skin from the sun

Everyone who has vitiligo can benefit from sun protection. Here's why:

1. Skin that has lost its color sunburns very easily.
2. A bad sunburn can worsen vitiligo.

Other Tips:

- Do not use tanning beds and sun lamps.
- Do not get a tattoo.
- Use sunscreen. Generously apply sunscreen every day to skin that will not be covered by clothing.

VOMITING

NATURAL HOME REMEDY

CLOVE & PEPPERMINT

HOW THE REMEDY WORKS

Vomiting is the forcible voluntary or involuntary emptying ("throwing up") of stomach contents through the esophagus and mouth. Vomiting can be caused by illness, excessive alcohol consumption; food poisoning and stomach disorders.

This clove and peppermint remedy helps to treat vomiting in the following ways:

1. **Clove:** Clove has antiseptic properties and fights many of the infections that cause vomiting while also calming the stomach.
2. **Peppermint:** Peppermint has a refreshing quality and naturally reduces vomiting and feelings of sickness.

HOW TO PREPARE THE REMEDY

1. Add 1 tablespoon of dried peppermint and 1 teaspoon of clove powder to a cup of hot water and let it steep for 5 minutes.
2. After 5 minutes, strain the water into another cup using a fine mesh strainer and drink it.
3. Drink this remedy up to 4 times per day until the vomiting subsides.

TIPS:

Try small amounts of clear liquids (water) stay hydrated.

- Drink Apple or cranberry juice
- Drink Chicken, beef or vegetable broth

Once food can be tolerated: To help replenish electrolytes that could be lost with vomiting eat foods and drink beverages that are rich in potassium and magnesium. Potassium-rich foods include bananas, potatoes, melons and tomatoes. Magnesium-rich foods include peanut butter and grains (breads, pastas, crackers, etc.).

Also See Remedy for Nausea in Part 3

WARTS

NATURAL HOME REMEDY

ALOE VERA & TEA TREE OIL

HOW THE REMEDY WORKS

Warts are a viral infection that causes rough, bumpy patches to appear on the skin. Common warts are an infection in the top layer of skin, caused by viruses in the human papillomavirus, or HPV, family. When the virus invades the outer layer of skin, usually through a tiny scratch, it causes rapid growth of cells on the outer layer of skin - creating the wart.

This aloe vera and tea tree oil remedy helps to treat warts in the following ways:

1. **Aloe Vera:** Aloe vera's anti-inflammatory properties soothe the skin affected by warts.
2. **Tea Tree Oil:** Tea tree oil is a powerful antiviral and directly targets the human papillomavirus (the virus that causes warts).

HOW TO PREPARE THE REMEDY

1. Place 1 teaspoon of aloe vera gel on a cotton ball and then massage it into the wart for 1 minute.
2. After 1 minute, add 5 drops of tea tree oil to a fresh cotton ball hold it over the wart and then use a bandage to hold it in place.
3. Replace the cotton ball and repeat this remedy 2 times per day until the wart is gone.

TIPS:

1. Because warts are caused by a virus, general immune system support can be effective in helping to keep warts from returning after treatment or to keep them from growing:
2. Eat a well balanced diet high in vitamins A, C, and E to help strengthen the immune system. Avoiding stress also help support a strong immune system.
3. Remember the viruses are more likely to cause warts when they come in contact with skin that is damaged or cut - don't bite your fingernails.

WHOOPING COUGH

NATURAL HOME REMEDY

ALMOND OIL CYPRESS OIL & EUCALYPTUS OIL

HOW THE REMEDY WORKS

Whooping cough (also known as pertussis) is a contagious bacterial disease. Many people think of whooping cough as a childhood disease, but it can strike people of any age. It causes uncontrollable violent coughing and also makes it difficult to breathe which leads to a whooping sound. When an infected person sneezes or coughs, tiny droplets containing the bacteria move through the air, and the disease is easily spread from person to person. The Initial symptoms are similar to the common cold and usually develop about a week after exposure to the bacteria.

This cypress oil and eucalyptus oil natural remedy helps to treat whooping cough in the following ways:

1. **Almond Oil:** Almond oil is a natural pain reliever and can soothe many of the symptoms associated with whooping cough.

2. **Cypress Oil:** Cypress oil is highly beneficial for the respiratory system and can eliminate whooping cough.
3. **Eucalyptus Oil:** Eucalyptus oil promotes proper breathing and enhances the recovery time for whooping cough.

HOW TO PREPARE THE REMEDY

1. Add 2 tablespoons of almond oil, 5 drops of cypress oil and 5 drops of eucalyptus oil to a bowl, mix well and then apply the mixture to your chest.
2. Use this remedy up to 2 times per day until the whooping cough subsides.

TIPS:

Whooping cough is highly contagious - and dangerous for newborns. Check with your healthcare provider for vaccine information. Make sure you and your family is protected.

Repeat: Whooping cough is spread by coughing and sneezing while in close contact with others, who then breathe in the whooping cough bacteria.

Practicing good hygiene is always recommended to prevent the spread of respiratory illnesses:

- Cover your mouth and nose with a tissue when you cough or sneeze.
- Put your used tissue in the waste basket.

- If you don't have a tissue, cough or sneeze into your upper sleeve or elbow, not your hands.
- Wash your hands often with soap and water for at least 20 seconds.
- If soap and water are not available, use an alcohol-based hand rub.

WORMS

NATURAL HOME REMEDY

COCONUT & PUMPKIN SEEDS

HOW THE REMEDY WORKS

Worms (also known as intestinal worms) are parasites that live on the intestinal wall. Some common causes of intestinal worms:

- Eating contaminated food.
- Drinking contaminated water.
- Poor sanitation/Poor personal hygiene.
- Using human excretion as fertilizer
- Eating raw and uncooked meat.

This coconut and pumpkin seeds remedy helps to treat worms in the following ways:

1. **Coconut:** Coconut contains various anti-parasitic ingredients that help to kill intestinal worms.
2. **Pumpkin Seeds:** Pumpkin seeds contain cucurbitacin - a compound that paralyzes worms and removes them from the intestinal wall.

HOW TO PREPARE THE REMEDY

1. Eat 1 tablespoon of dried, shredded coconut and 1 tablespoon of pumpkin seeds each morning shortly after waking up and then again each night shortly before you go to sleep.
2. Use this remedy daily until the worms disappear.

REMEDY VARIATION/TIPS:

Turmeric: Turmeric is an excellent home remedy for intestinal worms. Mix turmeric with water or butter milk. Dry powder or juice of turmeric mixed in butter milk or water is highly beneficial for intestinal problems.

- Add one tablespoon of turmeric juice to a glass of buttermilk or water. Drink it once daily for three consecutive days.

Eat **Carrots:** Carrots are very useful in treating worms; carrots can help clear worms quickly.

- Eat 3 small grated carrots on an empty every morning or drink carrot juice daily until the worms disappear.

Prevention: Preventing recurrence of Intestinal worms:

- Hygiene plays an important role in prevention of growth and transmission of intestinal worms. Brush teeth regularly
- Keeping nails short and get rid of nail biting habits in your child
- Wash hands with sanitizer before taking meal and after going to toilet.

WOUNDS

NATURAL HOME REMEDY

HONEY

HOW THE REMEDY WORKS

Honey is one of the oldest natural remedies for wounds and was used as a topical treatment for infected wounds as early as 50 AD by the Greek physician Dioscorides. There are a number of reasons honey is so effective at helping wounds to heal:

1. **Honey** Is Antibacterial: Honey kills off the bacteria cells that often form on fresh wounds and inhibit the healing process which allows your body to repair the wound at an accelerated rate.
2. **Honey** Is An Anti-Inflammatory: Honey fights the inflammation that often comes with wounds and helps to reduce any associated soreness and swelling.
3. **Honey** Speeds up the Recovery Process: Studies have shown that honey stimulates the growth of fresh skin tissue on wounds and helps them to heal faster.

When using honey as a natural remedy for wounds, it's important to remember that not all types of honey are created equal. *Manuka honey and raw honey are 100% natural and a great choice for treating wounds.

Processed honeys on the other hand, contain large amounts of high fructose corn syrup which actually increases the risk of a wound getting infected and should not be applied to wounds.

*Manuka honey is a monofloral honey produced in New Zealand and Australia from the nectar of the manuka tree. The honey is commonly sold as an alternative medicine.

HOW TO PREPARE THE REMEDY

Honey works best when directly applied to wounds. To prepare a natural wound healing remedy with honey, follow the instructions below:

- Apply 1 oz. of honey to a 4 inch x 4 inch waterproof dressing. If a larger dressing is required, adjust the amount of honey accordingly.
- Place the dressing on the wound and secure it with a bandage.

TIPS:

For the best results with this natural wound remedy, replace the honey covered dressing daily. If the wound is seeping fluid, replace the honey covered dressing up to 3 times per day depending on the amount of fluid that the wound exudes.

For deeper wounds, you should also fill the wound with honey before applying the honey covered dressing. This will help the wound to close faster and increase the effectiveness of the honey covered dressing.

REMEDY VARIATIONS: **To speed up your wound recovery, you can also try using the following natural wound healing ingredients in conjunction with this honey covered dressing remedy:**

- **Chamomile:** Chamomile is packed full of phytonutrients that accelerate the body's healing processes. To heal your wound with chamomile and honey, soak a chamomile teabag in water, drain it, press it against the wound and secure it in place with the honey covered dressing.
- **Garlic:** Garlic contains a compound called allicin which has powerful antibacterial and antifungal properties and is highly effective at healing wounds. However, it can also be harmful to the skin if left in contact with it for too long. To enjoy garlic's wound healing benefits without damaging your skin, combine 3 cloves of crushed garlic with a cup of water and let it stand for 2 hours. Then use a clean cloth to wipe the wound with this mixture every time you change the honey covered dressing.
- **Lavender**: Lavender has been shown to stimulate tissue regeneration and reduces scarring. To heal your wound with lavender and honey, apply 2-4 drops of lavender oil directly to the wound before applying the honey covered dressing.
- **Tea Tree Oil:** Tea tree oil is one of the most effective natural remedies for repairing the skin. To heal your wounds with tea tree oil and honey, apply 2-4 drops of tea tree oil directly to the wound before applying the honey covered dressing.

WRINKLES

NATURAL HOME REMEDY

ALOE VERA & EXTRA VIRGIN OLIVE OIL

HOW THE REMEDY WORKS

Wrinkles are lines or folds that appear on the skin and cause it to sag. Aging and sun exposure are the two major causes of wrinkles. As we age, our skin naturally becomes less elastic and more fragile. Also factors, such as pollutants and smoking can contribute to wrinkling.

This aloe vera and extra virgin olive oil remedy helps to treat wrinkles in the following ways:

1. **Aloe Vera:** Aloe vera boosts the elasticity of your skin and reduces the appearance of wrinkles.
2. **Extra Virgin Olive Oil:** Extra virgin olive oil re-moisturizes the skin and provides it with beneficial antioxidants which help to prevent wrinkles.

HOW TO PREPARE THE REMEDY

1. Massage 1 tablespoon of aloe vera gel into your wrinkles and then leave it for 15 minutes.
2. After 15 minutes, massage 1 tablespoon of extra virgin olive oil into your wrinkles, leave it for 15 minutes and then wash it clean with warm water.
3. Use this remedy up to 2 times per day to treat wrinkles.

REMEDY VARIATIONS/TIPS:

Eat Spinach: and other green leafy vegetables are good because it contains lutein that helps give the skin its essential antioxidant mechanism by maintaining skin hydration and elasticity. Ideally, you should eat about 10mg of this daily which is about 4oz of this vegetable.

Eat Goji berries: Goji berries are rich in Vitamin C that will help fight free radicals that damage the skin. Believe it or not, they contain 500 times more Vitamin C per ounce than what you get from oranges. It also has antioxidants such as vitamin B1, B2, B6 and E as well as linoleic acid, an essential fat that plumps up the skin making it look smoother and younger.

Be sure to have regular facials as this is very effective in controlling wrinkles. You should also give yourself a facial massage as this helps increase blood circulation which results in the tightening of the muscles which reduces the fleshiness of the skin and restores your youthful look. When you do a facial massage, make sure you always start from the neck upwards using all your fingers and massaging rapidly in a circular motion, and end at the forehead. If there are wrinkles on the jaw, pinch the skin between your thumb and fingers.

XEROSTOMIA

NATURAL HOME REMEDY

PEPPERMINT & ROSEMARY

HOW THE REMEDY WORKS

Xerostomia (also known as dry mouth) is caused by a lack of saliva in the mouth. People get dry mouth when the glands in the mouth that make saliva are not working properly. Dry mouth or reduced saliva can be caused by a number of factors. According to the National Institute of Dental and Craniofacial Research (NIH) more than 400 medicines can cause the salivary glands to make less saliva. For example, medicines for high blood pressure and depression often cause dry mouth. Also the use of tobacco or alcohol can dry out the mouth.

This peppermint and rosemary remedy helps to treat xerostomia in the following ways:

1. **Peppermint:** Peppermint increases saliva production and protects against dry mouth.
2. **Rosemary:** Rosemary moisturizes the mouth and stops it from drying out.

HOW TO PREPARE THE REMEDY

1. Add 1 tablespoon of dried peppermint and 1 tablespoon of dried rosemary to a cup of hot water and let it steep for 5 minutes.
2. After 5 minutes, strain the water into another cup using a fine mesh strainer and drink it.
3. Drink this remedy up to 4 times per day to treat dry mouth.

TIPS:

- Chew sugarless gum or suck on sugarless hard candy to stimulate saliva flow; citrus, cinnamon or mint-flavored candies are good choices.

- Sip water or sugarless drinks often.

- Avoid drinks with caffeine, such as coffee, tea, and some sodas. Caffeine can dry out the mouth.

Remember: Dry mouth is not a normal part of aging. If you have a dry mouth all or most of the time, it can be uncomfortable and can lead to serious health problems. See your dentist or healthcare provider to rule out any health problems.

YEAST INFECTION

NATURAL HOME REMEDY

MANUKA HONEY & YOGURT

HOW THE REMEDY WORKS

Yeast infections (also known as Candida) are a type of infection caused by microscopic yeast that can affect the breasts, nail beds and vaginal area. Yeast infections can be severely uncomfortable, itching, irritation and redness is but a few symptoms. Women have a greater risk of being diagnosed with having yeast infection due to estrogen levels, even though men have the potential of becoming infected as well.

Other possible causes of yeast infections include detergents, fabric softeners, feminine and hygiene sprays, and forms of contraceptives like foams or jellies. Menopause might also trigger the growth of the bacteria. In menopause, the estrogen levels drop which results to the thinning of the vaginal wall making it more susceptible to different kinds of organisms which could lead to various infections, including but not limited to yeast.

This manuka honey and yogurt remedy helps to treat yeast infections in the following ways:

1. **Manuka Honey:** Manuka honey fights the inflammation caused by yeast infections and alleviates many of their unpleasant symptoms.
2. **Yogurt:** Probiotic yogurt inhibits the growth of the yeast which causes infections.

HOW TO PREPARE THE REMEDY

1. Add 1 teaspoon of manuka honey to 1 cup of probiotic yogurt, mix it well and then eat it.
2. Use this remedy up to 4 times per day until the yeast infection subsides.

TIPS:

Diet: A good diet to treat yeast infection is a necessary step in the general treatment of the infection. It is also important to eat food that is fresh. It would be best to void processed and highly fatty foods, not only for your yeast infection but for your general health as well.
Eat a lot of garlic: Garlic contains antibacterial properties which help in eliminating the overgrowth of yeast. Also, *fresh ginger* can be a good condiment for yeast. Be generous with eating fresh greens. Steamed and sautéed would be the ideal cooking preparations. Try to avoid eating sweet vegetables like carrots, corn, potatoes, onions, and sweet potatoes.
Limit your intake of meat: Fish, beef, lamb, poultry and eggs are okay in moderation. It has been suggested that an ideal serving of meat should be no larger than half the size of your palm.

ZINC POISONING

NATURAL HOME REMEDY

LEMON JUICE & MILK

HOW THE REMEDY WORKS

Zinc poisoning is a rare but potentially harmful condition. Your risk for zinc poisoning can be due to a variety of factors. Not all people with risk factors will get zinc poisoning. Risk factors for zinc poisoning include:

- Excessive consumption of zinc supplements or a daily diet that exceeds recommended daily requirements.
- Exposure to toxic chemicals including paint, lead, industrial chemicals and cleaners, solvents, rubber, metal fumes, varnish, and antirust products.

Some common symptoms of zinc poisoning include: aches and pain, a persistent metal taste in the mouth, fever, and diarrhea, difficulty breathing, rash, and vomiting.

This lemon juice and milk remedy helps to treat zinc poisoning in the following ways:

1. **Lemon Juice:** The citric acid in lemon juice reacts with excess zinc and allows it to be removed from the body more easily.

2. **Milk:** Milk lines the stomach and helps to flush excess zinc out of your system.

HOW TO PREPARE THE REMEDY

1. Add 1 tablespoon of lemon juice to a glass of milk, mix it well and then drink it.
2. Drink this remedy up to 2 times per day to treat zinc poisoning.

WARNING:

Seek immediate medical help for serious symptoms, such as vomiting, seizure, inability to urinate, low blood pressure or difficulty breathing.

CALL POISON CONTROL, OR A LOCAL EMERGENCY NUMBER

In the United States, call 1-800-222-1222 to speak with a local poison control center (American Association of Poison Control Center). This hotline number will let you talk to experts in poisoning. They will give you further instructions.
This is a free and confidential service. All local poison control centers in the United States use this national number.

You should call if you have any questions about poisoning or poison prevention. You can call 24 hours a day, 7 days a week.
www.aapcc.org

ALPHABETICAL LIST OF INGREDIENTS

FOOD HERBS AND OILS

Here's an alphabetical checklist of Food, Herbs and Oils used in this book to help treat any aliments/illness you may suffer from. You may already have many of these ingredients in your home right now! Also you can find them at your local grocery or health food stores.

ALMOND OIL

- Back Pain
- Restless Leg Syndrome
- Whooping Cough

ALOE VERA GEL

- Gum Disease
- Oily Hair
- Warts
- Wrinkles

APPLE

- Oily Skin
- Energy

APPLE CIDER VINEGAR

- Acid Reflux
- Ear Infection
- Gallstones
- Kidney Stones
- Oral Thrush
- Psoriasis
- Upset Stomach

AVOCADO

- Frizzy Hair

BAKING SODA

- Acid Reflux
- Gas
- Rashes
- Urinary Tract Infection

BAKUCHI OIL

- Vitiligo

BANANA

- Dry Scalp
- Stomach Ulcers

BARLEY

- Jaundice

BASIL

- Fever
- Itching
- Menstrual Cramps
- Vertigo

BASIL OIL

- Fatigue
- Bitter Gourd
- Diabetes

BLACK PEPPER

- Toothache

BLACK TEA

- Cold Sores
- Oily Hair

CALENDULA

- Conjunctivitis

CARAWAY SEEDS

- Bloating

CARDAMOM

- Depression
- Sore Throat

CARROT

- Erectile Dysfunction
- Teething

CAT' S CLAW

- Inflammation

CAYENNE

- Back Pain
- Common Cold
- Coughs
- High Blood Pressure

- Tendonitis

CHAMOMILE

- Sleep Problems

CHAMOMILE OIL

- Anxiety
- Nerve Pain

CHASTEBERRY

- Menopause

CINNAMON

- Acne
- Diabetes
- Gas
- Menopause and Sore Throat

CLOVE

- Nausea
- Vomiting

CLOVE OIL

- Cramps

COCONUT

- Worms

COCONUT MILK

- Stomach Ulcers

COCONUT OIL

- Burns
- Chapped Lips
- Dandruff
- Hypothyroidism
- Rashes
- Vitiligo

COLLOIDAL OATMEAL

- Eczema
- Psoriasis

CORIANDER SEEDS

- Indigestion
- Vertigo

CORNSTARCH

- Diaper Rash

CRANBERRY JUICE

- Urinary Tract Infection

CUCUMBER

- Dry Eyes
- Oily Skin

CUMIN SEEDS

- Nausea

CYPRESS OIL

- Whooping Cough

DANDELION

- Fibroids

EPSOM SALT

- Eczema
- Edema

EUCALYPTUS OIL

- Asthma
- Fatigue
- Migraines
- Runny Nose
- Whooping Cough

EXTRA VIRGIN OLIVE OIL

- Dandruff/Dry Skin
- Ear Infection
- Lice
- Tendonitis
- Wrinkles

FENNEL SEEDS

- Bad Breath
- Bloating
- Indigestion
- Menstrual Cramps
- Queasiness

FENUGREEK SEEDS

- Common Cold

FIGS

- Constipation

FLAX SEEDS

- Constipation
- Irritable Bowel Syndrome

GARLIC

- Cold Sores
- Shingles
- Sinus Infection
- Toothache

GINGER

- Arthritis
- Bronchitis
- Fever
- Flu
- Hypothyroidism
- Jaw Pain
- Jet Lag
- Morning Sickness
- Queasiness
- Upset Stomach

GINKGO BILOBA

- Pre-Menstrual Syndrome

GRAPEFRUIT OIL

- Edema

GREEN TEA

- Blackheads
- Inflammation

ICE

- Cramps
- Neck Pain

LAVENDER OIL

- Anxiety
- Asthma
- Dry Eyes
- Eczema
- Headaches
- Neck Pain
- Restless Leg Syndrome

LEMON BALM

- Pre-Menstrual Syndrome

LEMON JUICE

- Acne
- Bad Breath
- Common Cold/Flu
- High Blood Pressure
- Jaundice/Jet Lag
- Morning Sickness
- Pimples
- Zinc Poisoning

LICORICE

- Shingles

LIME OIL

- Nasal Congestion

MANUKA HONEY

- Acid Reflux
- Acne
- Bronchitis
- Common Cold
- Flu
- Frizzy Hair
- Yeast Infection

MARJORAM OIL

- Nerve Pain

MATCHA GREEN TEA

- Energy

MILK

- Arthritis
- Chapped Lips
- Coughs
- Dry Skin
- Insomnia
- Stomach Ulcers

- Zinc Poisoning

MILK THISTLE

- Fibroids

NEEM OIL

- Ringworm

NETTLE LEAF

- Allergies
- Joint Pain

NUTMEG

- Insomnia

ORANGE OIL

- Nervousness

OREGANO OIL

- Sinus Infection

PASSIFLORA

- Obsessive Compulsive Disorder

PEPPERMINT

- Allergies
- Gallstones
- Heartburn
- Morning Sickness/Vomiting
- Xerostomia

PEPPERMINT OIL

- Migraines
- Snoring

POMEGRANATE JUICE

- Erectile Dysfunction

PUMPKIN SEEDS

- Worms

RAW POTATO

- Burns

RED CLOVER

- Hot Flashes

ROSE PETALS

- Chapped Lips

ROSEMARY

- Xerostomia

ROSEMARY OIL

- Headaches
- Nervousness
- Runny Nose

SAGE

- Hot Flashes

SEA SALT

- Gum Disease
- Toothache

SESAME SEED OIL

- Dry Scalp

SLIPPERY ELM

- Heartburn

SPINACH

- Energy

ST JOHN'S WORT

- Depression
- Jaw Pain
- Nerve Pain
- Obsessive Compulsive Disorder

ST JOHN'S WORT OIL

- Nerve Pain

TEA TREE OIL

- Blackheads
- Nasal Congestion
- Oral Thrush

- Pimples
- Ringworm
- Snoring
- Vaginal Infection
- Warts

TURMERIC

- Arthritis
- Coughs
- Joint Pain

VALERIAN

- Sleep Problems

WATERMELON

- Kidney Stones

WHEATGRASS JUICE

- Kidney Stones

WHITE VINEGAR

- Diaper Rash
- Lice

YOGURT

- Irritable Bowel Syndrome
- vaginal Infection
- Yeast Infection

"Even when all is known, the care of a man is not yet complete, because eating alone will not keep a man well; he must also take exercise. For food and exercise, while possessing opposite qualities, yet work together to produce health."

Hippocrates

WHY EAT ORGANIC FOODS

EATING ORGANIC

Organic foods have become very popular because of their offered health benefits. However, knowing the maze of organic food benefits and labels claims can be confusing. In fact, there are many people who asked if organic foods are really healthier or not. Why should you consider organic foods? Are they beneficial to your health? Well, whatever your questions are, it is important to know about organic foods.

Organic foods, as its name implies, are produced through organic farming. Nowadays, many countries promote organic farming as more and more people are seeking for organic foods that would provide them long-term health benefits.

Healthy eating can offer you a healthier life, which can help you, fight diseases and other health risks. But, for you to achieve this, you should eat more vegetables, fruits, good fats, and whole grains. However, some have questions about the safety, sustainability and nutrition of organic foods. So, what does organic means?

Organic Foods

Organic refers to the process on how products are produced and grown. Particular requirements should be maintained and met so that products will be labeled as organic. The organic crops should be grown in safe soil. They should have no modifications and should remain separate from the conventional products.

When it comes to producing organic foods, farmers are forbidden to use bioengineered genes or GMOs, synthetic pesticides, sewage fertilizers, and petroleum-based fertilizers. In terms of organic livestock, they should have access to outdoors and must be given organic feed. They will not be given growth hormones, antibiotics or any by- products.

What are GMOs or Genetically Modified Organisms?

GMOs or GE foods are animals or plants in which their DNA has been changed. Such products have undergone tests to know their effects on the environment and humans. In several countries, organic products don't intentionally contain GMOs.

The Benefits of Organic Foods

Organic foods offer a wide range of benefits. Several studies show that the organic foods have more beneficial nutrients than the conventionally grown foods. Moreover, people who have allergies to preservatives, chemicals or foods often seek for their symptoms to be reduced when they only eat organic foods. Aside from that, the best thing about organic foods is that they contain lesser pesticides. These pesticides are chemicals including herbicides, insecticides, and fungicides. Such chemicals are used in the conventional agriculture and the residues remain in or on the food you eat.

Understanding the Organic Food Labels

Once you have considered organic foods, there are several terms that you should understand in order for you to make the most of these foods. When shopping around, keep in mind that natural foods are not equivalent to organic foods. Natural foods don't have any production standards that must be met. This indicates that the food is not one hundred percent organic. There are also other labels offered on the organic foods in other countries like Canada and Australia. So, depending on your residency, make sure that you know the organic food labels for you to ensure that you are getting the right food.

No matter what type of diet you are into, organic foods should be your priority. Considering organic foods is an effectual option for planetary and personal health. Purchasing organically grown foods that are free from harmful chemicals and bursting with more taste and nutrition should be considered by all people across the globe as this can be the key for them to have good health. There are many reasons why you should switch to organic foods today, these are as follows:

Top Reasons Why You Should Eat Organic Foods:

Avoid Chemicals

Eating organic foods is the only key for you to avoid any harmful chemicals that are present on commercially grown foods. Over six hundred active chemicals were registered for agricultural use in the US and billions of pounds were used every year. However, because of organic farming, using such chemical was reduced and was only used on conventional foods. That is the reason why you can be assured that you are safer with organic foods.

Benefits from More Nutrients

Organic foods have higher content of beneficial nutrients compared to other foods. These foods contain nutrients including mineral, micronutrients, vitamins, and enzymes. The reason behind it is that the soil used is nourished and managed with sustainable practices by production standards. So, expect that you will get more nutrients once you have considered organic foods.

Better Taste

The best thing about organic foods is that they taste better because well-balanced and nourished soil produces strong and healthy plants. This is true with the heirloom varieties that are cultivated for the taste over appearance.

Avoid GMO

Foods that are genetically engineered are actually contaminating today's food supply. Therefore, if you want to make sure that your foods are healthy, choose only organic foods.

Avoid Antibiotics, Drugs, and Hormones in Animal Products

Conventional dairy and meat products contain highest risk for contamination. More than ninety percent of pesticides were consumed to product dairy and meat products. However, if you choose organic foods, you will be able to avoid this. Plus, you will get the right nutrients you deserve without indulging any chemicals or preservatives.

Lessen Pollution and Protects Soil and Water

Agricultural pesticides, fertilizers, and chemicals are contaminating in the environment, which poisons the supply of water and destroys the fertile farmland's value. The organic standards don't permit the utilization of toxic chemicals in farming and need responsible management of biodiversity and healthy soil.

Safe and Healthy

Organic foods have the power to help you keep safe and healthy. According to some experts, organic foods can prolong one's life and can offer a healthier lifestyle. So, if you want to get rid of any diseases or some health risks, then this is the right time for you to stay healthy by considering organic foods.

Note: Determine If the Food is Natural or Organic

When shopping around, it is important to determine if your foods you chose are natural or organic. You have to keep in mind that natural is different from organic.

Natural foods may be partly organic and partly not. The reason behind it is that natural foods do not meet any standards in organic farming. But, once food is stated organic foods, they are produced in accordance to the standards set by a particular country. So, make sure that your chosen food is organic not natural as this can make a difference.

See the Shopper's Guide on next page ~The Most Important Produce To Buy Organic.

The Environmental Working Group (EWG) is an American environmental organization that specializes in research and advocacy in the areas of toxic chemicals, agricultural subsidies, public lands, and corporate accountability. (Wikipedia)

According to EWG the following "Dirty Dozen Plus" had the highest pesticide load, making them the most important to buy organic.

PRODUCE TO BUY ORGANIC

12 THE DIRTY DOZEN - USE THIS GUIDE

1. Apples
2. Celery
3. Cherry Tomatoes
4. Cucumbers
5. Grapes
6. Nectarines (imported)
7. Peaches
8. Potatoes
9. Snap peas (imported)
10. Spinach
11. Strawberries
12. Sweet bell peppers

Plus - EWG characterizes as "highly toxic" and of special concern:

1. Hot Peppers
2. Kale/Collard Greens

15 CLEAN FOODS - USE THIS GUIDE

According to EWG's research, of the fruit and vegetable categories tested, the following "Clean 15" foods had the lowest pesticide load, and consequently are the safest conventionally grown crops to consume from the standpoint of pesticide contamination:

1. Asparagus
2. Avocados
3. Cabbage
4. Cantaloupe (domestic)
5. Cauliflower
6. Eggplant
7. Grapefruit
8. Kiwi
9. Mangoes
10. Onions
11. Papayas
12. Pineapples
13. Sweet Corn
14. Sweet Peas (frozen)
15. Sweet Potatoes

NOTE: It is always best to buy and eat organic whenever possible, including the 15 clean foods listed above.
The Environmental Working Group (EWG) is a nonprofit organization that advocates for policies that protect global and individual health. **www.ewg.org**

SUMMARY

BE SAFE: If you are taking any prescription drugs - If you are pregnant or breast-feeding, always talk with your doctor or healthcare provider before taking any herbal remedies. This also applies to giving herbal remedies to children... **SAFETY FIRST!**

"All that man needs for health and healing has been provided by God in nature, the challenge of science is to find it."

PHILIPPUS THEOPHRASUS

ABOUT THE AUTHOR

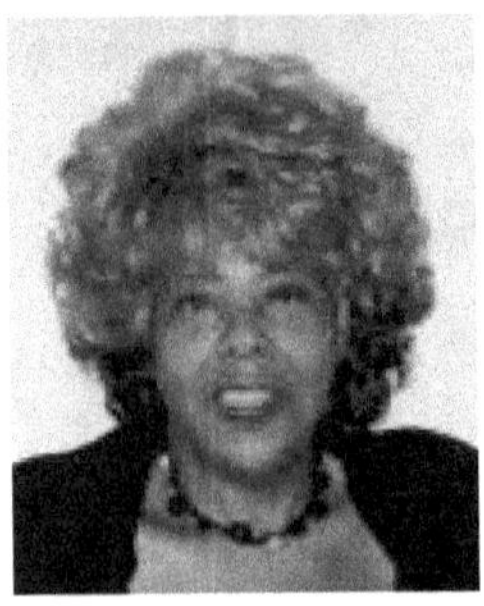

Hello, my name is Yvonne P. Johnson. I am a Board Certified Holistic Health Coach, with a passion for helping people become more aware of the prize of good health.

My mission is to teach and engage people in taking control of their lifestyle everyday (starting with good nutrition). Understanding and practicing good health is a top priority in life and when practiced you can prove that good health truly is your wealth.

Discover for yourself the Health and Wealth Connection. Be Wealthy Be Healthy Believe!

Thank you for purchasing my book.
I sincerely hope this book has proved useful to you and allows you to naturally treat any ailments/illness that you suffer from. For more information on Life Changing Health and Fitness Issues ~ please visit my websites at:

www.bewealthybehealthybelieve.com
www.fitbodyandmore.com

To Your Prosperity!

Yvonne P. Johnson, HHC

www.ingramcontent.com/pod-product-compliance
Lightning Source LLC
Chambersburg PA
CBHW070852290526
45795CB00001B/84

* 9 7 8 1 5 1 1 9 8 6 1 0 6 *